50 THINGS THAT CAUSE ACNE

Inara Hasanali

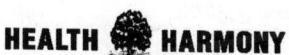

An imprint of
B. Jain Publishers (P) Ltd.
USA — Europe — India

Disclaimer

Any information given in this book is not intended to be taken as a replacement for medical advice. Any person with a condition requiring medical attention should consult a qualified practitioner or therapist.

50 THINGS THAT CAUSE ACNE

First Edition: 2011
1st Impression: 2011

All rights reserved. No part of this book may be reproduced, stored in a retrieval system or transmitted, in any form or by any means, mechanical, photocopying, recording or otherwise, without any prior written permission of the publisher.

© with author

Published by Kuldeep Jain for

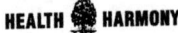

An imprint of
B. JAIN PUBLISHERS (P) LTD.
1921/10, Chuna Mandi, Paharganj, New Delhi 110 055 (INDIA)
Tel.: +91-11-4567 1000 • *Fax:* +91-11-4567 1010
Email: info@bjain.com • *Website:* **www.bjain.com**

Printed in India by
J.J. Offset Printers

ISBN: 978-81-319-1137-2

Foreword

Acne forms the bulk of my dermatology practice. Over a few decades I have watched anxious parents usher their children into the clinic seeking a quick fix for the zits that dot the faces of their teenagers like a landmine. In today's cyber-world, they come armed with knowledge in all its phases of evolution from the ancient myths to the latest state of the art treatment. Some ask about the cause of acne and a few ask about the preventive measures that could reduce the flares that accompany acne leading to mutilating scars.

Acne is a chronic inflammation of the pilo-sebaceous glands with a curious multi-factorial aetiology. Treatment would therefore be effective if all the causes are addressed at all levels, be it hygiene, food, hormones, drugs, stress or myths. Inara Hasanali has, with her years of experience as a nutritionist, researched the possible culprit foods that have been linked to acne and the flares that accompany acne. The formidable food list attempts to create a level of awareness. Its usage has to be coupled with a food challenge diary over a period of time, in which a meticulous record is maintained to show an increase in acne or a flare of acne with the inclusion or exclusion of a particular food along the lines of a "who-dun-it".

This book is not a substitute for treatment with a specialist; however, it will be an eye-opener to people suffering from acne, especially those on long term antibiotic intervention. If used with realistic expectations from a preventive perspective, it will certainly help towards the effective treatment of acne and the mutilating scars they can form if left unattended.

Dr Susie Samuel
MBBS, DGO, Dip. Derm (London)
Fortis Malar Hospital, Chennai

Preface

"The best six doctors anywhere
And no one can deny it
Are sunshine, water, rest, and air
Exercise and diet.
These six will gladly you attend
If only you are willing
Your mind they'll ease
Your will they'll mend
And charge you not a shilling."

Nursery Rhyme quoted by Wayne Fields, **What the River Knows** 1990

I have always believed that the above six factors are essential for a healthy mind and body not when I was a child since I had not learnt this nursery rhyme in my childhood but from adolescence when I first began my long and interesting journey with food as an undergraduate student of nutrition.

By writing this book on acne, I have once again realised how important a balanced diet is to maintain health. The skin manifests the imbalances in the body. The causes of these imbalances are many and perhaps some of these imbalances are the causes of acne.

I have also found that generally acne is not the result of one cause. It can be due to multiple causes. It is also quite an individualistic condition. It does cause a certain amount of trauma during adolescence, but perhaps it is worse when it continues through adulthood.

In today's modern world there is a plethora of treatments available for acne. Being patient, living a simple life, following those six doctors mentioned above and being stress free may just be the best cure for mild and even moderate cases of acne. However, for severe cases it is absolutely essential to follow the advice of qualified dermatologists.

Some simple treatments have been laid out in this book for an individual to follow but always remember–although all of us would like to cure the conditions we suffer from by ourselves, without consulting specialists, if things start going mildly wrong it is better to consult specialists, rather than wait too long and consult them at the last moment.

With and without treatment, acne generally fades away as adolescents become adults. However, in this world where self-esteem is sometimes linked to clear skin and other extraneous factors, there are alternatives available to treat the condition. Please treat your acne breakouts for the following two reasons: The first being that the condition bothers you psychologically and the second being that non-treatment is making the acne worse.

There are treatments available but there is no 'one size fits all treatment' available. Researchers have formed no conclusions on the exact causes or the correct treatments for acne. Do try the treatments that suit you and discard the ones that don't suit you. Always remember to ask for specialists help if the situation worsens.

Inara Hasanali

Acknowledgements

I am extremely grateful to the Almighty and the universe for all the blessings showered on me.

I am also grateful for the support of my parents Soghra and Hasanali, my siblings: My sisters who are my greatest ever support—Yasmin, Nasreen, Parveen and my brother Sajjad. I also thank the numerous uncles, aunties (especially Salma Aunty), brothers-in-laws, cousins, nieces and nephews for their encouragement.

I thank the entire team at B Jain Publications, especially Mr. Nitin Jain, Dr. Geeta Rani Arora and the rest of the team who have been involved and have helped in publishing this book. A special thanks to the gracious Ms. Nina Kochhar for being kind enough to introduce me to my publishers.

Many friends have always stood by me but some of them have overextended themselves to support me through this book. A deeply felt grateful thanks to Bob Thompson for his quiet and constant support through all the different phases I have gone through writing this book, Sherwin Rodrigues for his encouragement and support from the beginning to the end of the book, Padma Sundareson for reading the manuscript and offering valuable suggestions, especially for the glossary and Nic Hallac for her words of encouragement and her faith in my creativity.

I would also like to thank all the researchers and acne sufferers who shared their knowledge with me.

God bless all of you.

Publisher's Note

"50 things that cause Acne" is the first book in our new series of books that we are launching. The name of "50 things" will be the common denominator or factor in this series as we will discuss 50 things that cause various common ailments.

In these books all the possible etiologies of the ailments will be discussed which, if taken care of, may keep the diseases at bay .The books in the series will also have the do's and don'ts for the condition discussed. The different treatment forms available are and will also be covered in brief.

The concept of these pocket books is to cover basic information about the disease and its causative factors. This can help a person to avoid the triggering factors and have an easier life and a more healthy and active life.

The author of this book is Inara Hasanali. She has been a writer since many years .She has done extensive research to give this project a shape and structure. It has been a pleasure working with such an author who is so meticulous. We hope you find the information in this book useful for keeping Acne at bay.

Kuldeep Jain
C.E.O., B. Jain Publishers (P) Ltd.

Contents

Foreword .... *iii*
Preface .... *v*
Acknowledgements .... *ix*
Publisher's Note .... *xi*

Chapters

1. Introduction 1
2. What is Acne? 5
3. What are the Various Types of Acne? 9
4. Grades or Types of Acne 23
5. Causes of Acne 25
   Alcohol 26
   Bacteria 29
   Caffeine 31
   Cosmetics 33
   Dirt 34
   Drugs 35

Artificial Sweeteners	39
Baker's Yeast	40
Beef	41
Broccoli	43
Candy	45
Cheese	47
Chocolate	48
Corn	50
Cream	51
Eggs	52
Garlic	54
Gluten	55
Ice cream	57
Lamb	58
Mangoes	59
Margarine	61
Milk	62
Mushroom	64
Oysters	66
Peanuts	68
Pickles	70
Pineapple	71
Potatoes	72
Refined Wheat Flour	73

	Rice	74
	Ready Meals	75
	Sesame	77
	Soy or Soya Milk	78
	Spelt	80
	Spicy Food	81
	Sugars	83
	Tuna	85
	Trans Fats	86
	Walnut	88
	Wheat Bran	90
	Wheat Germ	92
	Wheat Flour	93
	Genetics	95
	Hormones	97
	Occupation	99
	Pressure	101
	Smoking	102
	Stress	104
	Vitamin Deficiency	106
6.	Treatment of Acne	109
	Antibiotics	109
	Anti-inflammatories	111
	Benzoyl Peroxide	112

Dermabrasion	114
Hormonal Treatment	116
Intralesional Corticosteroid Injections	118
Laser	119
Phototherapy	120
Retinoids	122
Oral	123
Salicylic Acid	125
Sulphur	126
Surgery	127
Other Treatments	128
Aromatherapy	132
Ayurvedic Treatment for Acne	133
Azelaic Acid	133
Black Currant Seed Oil	134
Chinese Herbal Medicine	135
Cod Liver Oil	135
Evening Primrose Oil	136
Flaxseed Oil	137
Homoeopathy	137
Lemon Juice and Cucumber	138
Olive Leaf Extract	139
Reflexology	139
Vitamins A, B_5 and E	140

	Vitamin E	141
	Yoga	141
	Zinc	143
7.	Management of Acne	145
	Management of Mild Acne	145
	Management for Moderate Acne	145
	Management for Severe Acne	146
	Management for Very Severe Acne	146
	Tips	147
	Certain Healthy Foods	152

Glossary   *157*

References   *167*

Chapter 1

Introduction

Did you know that according to statistics, over 90 per cent of the world's population has suffered from very mild if not moderate or severe acne at least once in their lifetime? It is indeed a large figure and a majority of human beings have suffered from the ignominy of getting at least one pimple, blackhead or whitehead either in their teenage and adolescent years or sometimes in their twenties, thirties, forties, even fifties and sixties.

Acne affects the skin of all races from different parts of the globe, living under different climatic and socio-economic conditions. It does not discriminate against any population except chronologically as it first manifests itself generally during the pre-pubertal and pubertal age when teens start getting their first unwanted spots, generally on their faces.

Through the ages, no cure has been found, as yet. However, many treatments that decrease the severity of acne, are available. Being such a common condition, there should have been a treatment to clear acne, but since the exact cause of acne has not yet been found there has been no cure for it. Different people get acne at different ages for various reasons. Many people find that they are able to treat their acne through various treatments though treatment may evade a few. Many cases of acne have cleared up as the individual grows out of adolescence and becomes an adult but sometimes the condition persists into adulthood and needs to be treated.

Generally, acne has no major complications. However, it causes psychological distress more than physical discomfort. In moderate and severe cases, the skin may get inflamed and this causes both physical and emotional distress. Despite there being no single method of treatment which suits everyone, there are various options to choose from. Though the time of cure may be long, acne is a treatable if not avoidable condition.

It is important to maintain a positive attitude and not give in to psychological trauma. It is difficult, especially during the teens to adjust to outbreaks and flare-ups of acne but balancing the lifestyle with the best possible treatment that suits the individual can decrease acne. Patience, an openness to try various treatments, building a good relationship with your dermatologist and persisting with treatments which may take time to show results go a long way in decreasing the symptoms if not curing acne.

Despite the fact that treating acne is not considered important by some, it is important as acne can cause distress and increase the anxiety levels, especially in adolescents who are already undergoing several changes during puberty. Controlling their acne breakouts may improve their self-esteem and decrease anxiety. It can also prevent further flare-ups and prevent the formation of scars which may result as acne proceed from mild to moderate and then to severe levels leading to the possibility of permanent scarring.

There are many questions about acne in one's mind. Here are some answers to the most common ones.

Chapter 2
What is Acne?

Acne is a term generally used to characterize a wide range of lesions, spots, pimples, zits and inflammations affecting the skin. The surface of human skin consists of innumerable pores. Each pore opens into a canal called the follicle. Each follicle has a hair and an oil gland. The function of the oil glands or sebaceous glands is to lubricate the skin and to remove old skin cells. This, whole unit is called a pilosebaceous unit. Sometimes, due to various causes, the oil glands secrete extra oil or sebum. Thus, the pores in the skin get blocked and debris, dirt

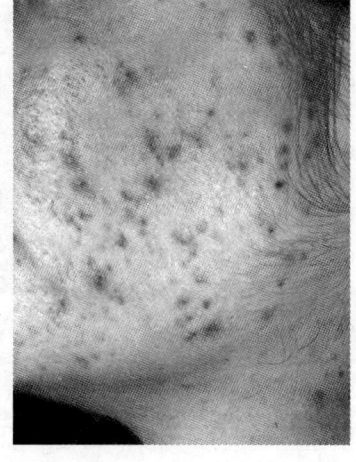

and bacteria accumulate in these enlarged pores. These pores are called plugs or comedones.

Acne is generally seen on the face, neck, back and shoulders of individuals due to the over-activity of sebaceous glands. It may be seen on others parts of the body sometimes. It may be present as either an inflammatory or a non-inflammatory condition.

Acne spots or blemishes are characterised as:
- Blackheads
- Whiteheads
- Papules
- Pustules
- Nodules
- Cysts

Blackheads are medically known as open comedones. They are seen as black or brownish bumps mainly on the nose. A blackhead is caused due to accumulation of sebum and not as a result of dirt 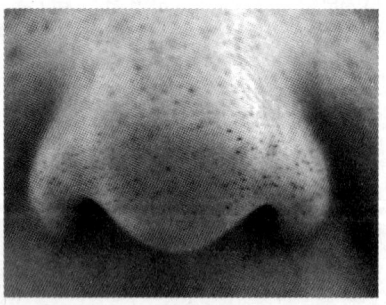 accumulation. It sometimes has a brownish appearance due to irregular light reflection from clogged hair follicles. It contains skin debris, oil and bacteria.

Whiteheads are closed comedones. A whitehead obstructs the skin opening and may burst open and cause inflammation in the surrounding skin.

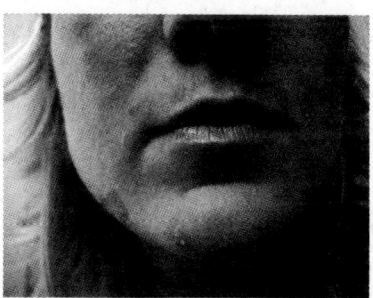

Papules are small, solid, rounded, raised, reddish spots on the skin. They may not contain any fluid and vary in size from being as small as a pinhead or reach a circumference of less than a centimetre.

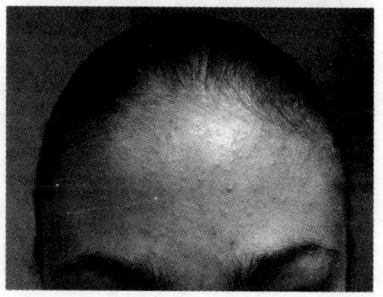

Pustules are small, inflamed elevations on the skin. They generally contain pus which is a combination white blood cells and cell debris.

Nodules are similar to papules but are larger, both in width and depth. They may be benign but are painful. They are generally over one centimeter wide.

Cysts are generally closed cavities formed in the skin. They are filled with liquid, semisolid or solid material. Cysts are the result of the inflammation going deep into the skin and affecting it. They are similar to nodules but may be smaller or bigger than them and always contain a fluid material. They are generally quite painful.

It is important to note that one should not squeeze nodules and cysts as they will worsen the condition and would further traumatize the skin.

Chapter 3
What are the Various Types of Acne?

There are various types of acne. They include:
- Acne vulgaris
- Acne rosacea
- Acne tropicalis
- Acne conglobata
- Acne fulminans
- Gram negative folliculitis
- Nodulocystic acne
- Pyoderma faciale
- Acne miliaris necrotica
- Infantile acne (neonatal acne)

- Excoriated acne
- Drug induced acne (steroid acne)
- Halogen acne
- Occupational acne (oil acne/tar acne)
- Acne cosmetica
- Acne aestivalis
- Acne keloidalis nuchae
- Acne mechanica
- Pomade acne
- Acne necrotica
- Lupus miliaris disseminatus faciei
- Acne with facial oedema

Acne Vulgaris

Acne vulgaris is the scientific term for the most common manifestation of acne, generally seen on the face, the back and the upper chest. It generally appears during puberty. When people suffer from acne, their pilosebaceous units are affected. The clinical symptoms include seborrhoea which is characterised by a scaly, reddish skin, or comedones—blackheads and whiteheads, papules or pinheads, pustules or pimples and nodules.

Although there is no single factor involved, multiple factors have been implicated as the cause of acne. Generally, acne is a result of over-activity of the sebaceous glands and hormonal changes during pre-puberty, puberty for both boys and girls, before menstruation, during pregnancy, pre-menopause and menopause for women. Genetics is also considered as important factor triggering outbreaks of acne. Acne may produce scarring in individuals.

Acne Rosacea

It is a chronic skin condition that affects adults. It generally affects adults between the ages of 30-60 years. It affects women more than men. Although more commonly seen in white Caucasian women, it also affects darker skinned people, where it is less easily diagnosed due to pigmentation.

Though it seems to be similar to acne it is not a form of acne. In this condition, blood vessels of the face expand, giving the face a flushed appearance. There is constant redness on the face, forehead and chin. The eyes may also get affected.

In severe cases, there may be red bumps or whiteheads or spots as well. It can be treated but not cured. It is advisable to contact a dermatologist and not to use over the counter topical medicines available for acne.

Acne Tropicalis

Tropical acne or acne tropicalis is a severe form of acne. In this condition, large nodules and pustules appear over various parts of the body including the neck, the back, the upper arms and the buttocks. The condition is aggravated by high temperatures and humidity, the sun and sweating. Hence, it is sometimes referred to as summer acne. It affects lighter skins more easily as they are unable to bear the tropical heat and humidity. Avoiding sunlight and over the counter topical remedies may work for mild cases but do contact a dermatologist if symptoms persist.

Acne Conglobata

This is a serious form of acne and is a chronic disease. It mainly affects men as it is associated with the androgen testosterone. The condition is inflammatory. It is characterized by the presence of comedones, nodules and abscesses. Nodules form around multiple comedones and increase in size till they finally burst discharging the pus in them into the surrounding skin. The skin get damaged and scarred due to the formation of cysts. It can be treated with the help of a dermatologist.

Acne Fulminans

This condition often develops after the unsuccessful treatment of acne conglobata. It has a sudden onset and is characterized by severe inflammation. It can be accompanied by fever and aching knee and hip joints. Please consult a dermatologist for treatment.

Gram Negative Folliculitis

In this condition follicles are inflamed by bacteria which may be resistant to several antibiotics. It may develop as a consequence of long term treatment with antibiotics. It is essential to contact a dermatologist to treat this condition.

Nodulocystic Acne

This type of acne is characterized by the formation of large painful cysts which may be several centimeters in width. The cysts are inflamed and filled with pus. They may be present singly or in clusters over the scalp, the face, the neck, the shoulders and the back.

It is important that a person does not drain the cysts on his own and consults a dermatologist to drain them and follows the treatment recommended by them.

Pyoderma Faciale

This unusual type of acne generally affects young women between the ages of 20–40 years, and is often mistaken for acne rosacea. It is also called rosacea fulminans. In this condition, the acne flares-up suddenly as pustules and nodules form all over the face. It is painful. There is no flushing of the skin and the eyes are not affected.

Since it is rare and its cause is unknown, it is advisable to consult a dermatologist and start treatment. According to some opinions, there may be a hormonal imbalance. Most cases of persons with this type of acne clear up after regular treatment.

Acne Miliaris Necrotica

This condition is also called **propioni bacterium folliculitis** or **scalp folliculitis**. Small, itchy and painful pustules are seen along the hairline or within the scalp. Though the exact cause is unknown *propionibacterium* acnes, certain yeasts and mites have been indicted.

Cleaning the scalp with a mild shampoo and the use of prescribed antibiotics or steroids are effective in treating this condition. It is advisable to reduce stress levels as some reports show that stress worsens this condition.

Infantile Acne or Neonatal Acne

Though it may be surprising to believe so, neonatal or infantile acne has been seen in some rare cases in newborn babies or infants between the ages of 6–16 months and has been documented. It may be the result of increased sebum production, hormonal factors or genetics. It may be present as blackheads, whiteheads, inflamed papules, pustules, nodules or cysts. One study showed that it is more predominant in male infants and responds quite well to various treatments depending upon the severity of acne. More studies are required to establish its exact cause and to find the best and most suitable treatment.

Excoriated Acne

It may be difficult for an acne prone individual to stop squeezing and picking at the comedones, papules and pustules present on their skin. Unfortunately, this makes one's acne condition worse and leads to the formation of red marks, irritated skin and permanent scarring. It is advisable to avoid picking or squeezing scars in front of a mirror. This compulsive urge to pick at, scratch or squeeze visible or invisible acne is called excoriated acne. Talking to a dermatologist and trying out the treatments suggested by them is a practical approach to solving this problem.

Drug Induced Acne or Steroid Acne

This acne is caused in individuals who have been prescribed steroids for some illnesses they suffer from and they unfortunately get acne as a side effect. Anabolic steroids have been implicated as a cause of acne. However, it should be noted that when used properly, steroids also treat important illnesses and perhaps misuse rather than prescribed use of steroids may be responsible for acne outbreaks. Sometimes the positive effects of prescribed steroids negate minor side effects like acne.

Some studies have shown that when steroids are prescribed to treat acne there is no rebound effect and the patients did not get perioral dermatitis or steroid acne after being treated with 0.75 per cent hydrocortisone and 0.5 per cent of precipitated sulphur.

Halogen Acne

Halogen acne is a condition that results when a sensitive individual ingests salts from the halogen family including chlorine, fluorine, bromine or iodine present in certain medicines or products containing any of these elements. Acne generally appears around the area surrounding the mouth and the chin. It is often mild and can be treated.

Exposure to compounds from the halogen family by those who work in such factories or pharmaceuticals has also been reported by various researchers. The presence of these compounds in the environment may trigger the acne. Non-occupational contamination due to industrial accidents, contaminated food products or even waste, has been documented in older studies in Asia.

Occupational Acne or Oil Acne or Tar Acne

Some occupations trigger or exacerbate the onset of acne in certain individuals. Certain oils including petroleum based oils and grease cause oil acne in individuals. In oil acne, the individual finds blisters or spots in areas most exposed to these oils. These areas include the arms and hands. However, other areas including the abdomen and thighs can also get affected due to oil stained clothes. It is important to consult a dermatologist and treat the condition so that it does not deteriorate further to cause other skin complications. Exposure to sun worsens the condition and causes the skin to darken.

Coal tar products can cause tar acne. In this condition, black plugs are found in individuals generally around the eyes. There may be skin darkening and the sufferers find that they experience burning sensations or flushing of skin or both when exposed to sunlight. As with oil acne, it is important to consult a dermatologist so that the condition is treated and does not create future skin complications.

Acne Cosmetica

It is a mild but persistent form of acne caused when your skin reacts to the use of certain cosmetics. Some individuals develop sensitivity to make up, sun blocks or lip products and this may cause acne or worsen existing acne. They may realize that the chemicals in these formulations clog the pores of their skin as their condition worsens after use of these cosmetics.

Though small pinkish-red bumps are seen all over the body, acne cosmetica commonly manifests itself on the face and arms. It is characterized by comedones and sometimes papules and pustules may also be produced. It is generally non-inflammatory. When it is mild, stopping the cosmetic or switching over to non-comedogenic products can help. If the condition persists, please consult a dermatologist.

Acne Aestivalis

This condition is also called **Mallorca Acne**. It is seen after natural sun exposure or exposure to UV light from tanning and manifests itself as red papular lesions. Outbreaks often start during summer and continue through other seasons. It rarely leaves scars behind but may continue for a long time.

When mild, several topical applications may be effective but in severe cases it requires the expertise of a dermatologist to treat and cure it.

Acne Keloidalis Nuchae

This condition is chronic and generally affects males. It is seen more often in men of African descent, followed by Hispanics and Asians when compared to other males. Papules and pustules occur mainly on the scalp and on the posterior neck. The lesions are often painful. Although it resembles acne lesions, it is not a form of acne.

The exact cause has not been isolated. There is scarring and it is advisable to consult a dermatologist to treat this condition.

Acne Mechanica

Acne mechanica is a condition where physical pressure, friction, or covered skin aggravated by heat causes acne. Many trigger factors have been identified. Some of them include helmets, tight shoulder pads, tight back straps, tight clothing, tight caps and musical instruments resting snuggly for hours together against the neck.

Try to decrease these causes, shower frequently, use natural fabrics and see if topical medicines decrease the acne. If symptoms of acne persist, don't forget to consult a dermatologist.

Pomade Acne

Pomades are thick oily dressings used to style hair. They are often used to straighten curly hair or to mould hair into different shapes. Pomades are easily available in many shops. Some people also make pomades at home. However they may be made, pomades can cause pomade acne in certain individuals. It is seen more often in darker rather than lighter coloured skin.

This acne generally affects regions such as the scalp, the forehead and the temples. It may erupt as multiple comedones, papules and pustules. Sometimes the skin in these regions gets inflamed. The best method available to avoid this acne is to stop using pomades and hope that the acne clears up naturally. Perhaps pomades can be used away from the scalp if they have to be used. If the acne does not clear up naturally, topical medication can be used. However, if this treatment does not work it is important to consult a dermatologist.

Acne Necrotica

Acne necrotica or **folliculitis necrotica** is generally seen in adult males. In this condition, several painful pustules, from the size of a pinhead up to the size of a pea are formed. These pustules are generally itchy, painful and inflamed. They may be found in the upper body prominently along the front hairline.

It is better to seek the help of a qualified dermatologist to treat the condition. As the dead cells necrotize and die, they leave behind deep depressed scars which need the help of a dermatologist. The exact cause of this condition is not known.

Lupis Miliaris Disseminatus Faciei

This skin condition is quite rare. Asians, more specifically Japanese and young men rather than young women may be more prone to get affected by this condition. It affects the face and the eyelids which get covered with dome shaped inflammatory lesions. Though it has been linked to acne rosacea by a few researchers, the exact cause is unknown. Red, brown and yellow-brown pustules appear singularly or in groups, mainly on the face, eyelids and sometimes the upper lip.

No specific treatment has been identified and it is better to consult a qualified dermatologist to cure the lesions and residual scars which form on the skin. According to researchers, it spontaneously resolves itself in a year or two making it difficult to assess the impact of different treatments.

Acne with Facial Oedema

Sometimes after the treatment of acne vulgaris, solid facial oedema may appear as a complication. This is quite a rare occurrence. Generally the swelling is treated by a dermatologist using oral steroids and isotretinoin and ketotifen. In rare cases, the swelling does not subside.

Chapter 4

Grades or Types of Acne

Many researchers have been involved in the grading of acne counting diverse lesions like comedones, papules, pustules, nodules and cysts. Some use physical examination, others use photographs, etc. However, till date there is no perfect global consensus but currently four grades are globally recognised. They are:

Grade I or Mild Acne

In mild acne the skin has comedones, mainly blackheads and whiteheads. A few papules may sometimes be present. Generally there is no inflammation and scarring.

Grade II or Moderate Acne

With moderate acne, the skin has comedones plus small papules. Sometimes a few pustules are also present. When mild acne is left untreated, it may lead to moderate acne. The skin gets inflamed and may require the services of a dermatologist.

Grade III or Severe Acne

This is a severe form of acne and often develops when moderate acne is left untreated. There are comedones, papules and pustules to be treated and it requires the services of a dermatologist. Sometimes a few nodules are also present.

Grade IV or Very Severe Acne

This is also called **cystic acne**. One can find papules, pustules, nodules and large cysts. It is a severe and painful condition. It is absolutely essential to be under the treatment of a qualified and experienced dermatologist.

Chapter 5
Causes of Acne

There is no single cause of teenage or adult acne. Many factors have been implicated. Many research studies have been conducted through the decades. Some of the below described causes have been proven to cause acne while the final verdict for some of the others causes is not yet out. However, it is important to remember that acne is an individualistic disease and just as one treatment may suit a specific individual, it may have absolutely no positive effect in treating the next individual. Different causes may be the reason why certain individuals are more prone to acne flare-ups when compared to others.

It is important to identify the cause to specifically treat acne. Sometimes elimination of possible causes also works; for example, by identifying specific food allergies which may not cause acne but may definitely exacerbate acne breakouts.

Another point to be noted is that although flare-ups or outbreaks of acne may be instant or within a period of 24 hours, most treatments take weeks to resolve the acne present in individuals.

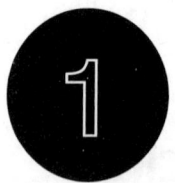

Alcohol

Drinking is a personal decision. Many people believe that alcohol relieves stress and makes them feel relaxed. Social drinking is a part and parcel of many civil societies. It is also a part of the lifestyle of some cultures.

Red wine forms a major part of the Mediterranean diet, a diet considered to be one of the healthiest ones on the planet. Moderate drinking has been a part of the diet of people from this region. However it must be noted that together with the wine, the diet is extremely rich in many protective foods including whole grains, olive oil and many servings of fruits and vegetables on a daily basis. There is also a certain amount of exercise in their lifestyle and all these factors contribute to the health benefits of the Mediterranean diet.

As with other causes, there are no specific research findings linking the consumption of alcohol with the outbreak of acne. However, there are a few research studies on the effect of alcohol on hormone levels. Heavy consumption of alcohol leads to an increase of both testosterone and oestrogen.

There are a few theories proposed including the hormone factor influencing acne. Others believe that alcohol may increase sebum production. As there is not enough research on the link of alcohol with acne, it not easy to draw a conclusion on its effects on acne. The effect may be more on an individualistic level or more pronounced in those who suffer from hormonal imbalances due to a variety of factors.

Alcohol has been implicated as a causative factor of many lifestyle diseases, being both a direct cause and an indirect one. When it becomes a causative factor as a promoter of conditions or diseases it is a good idea to consume it in moderation or to abstain from it.

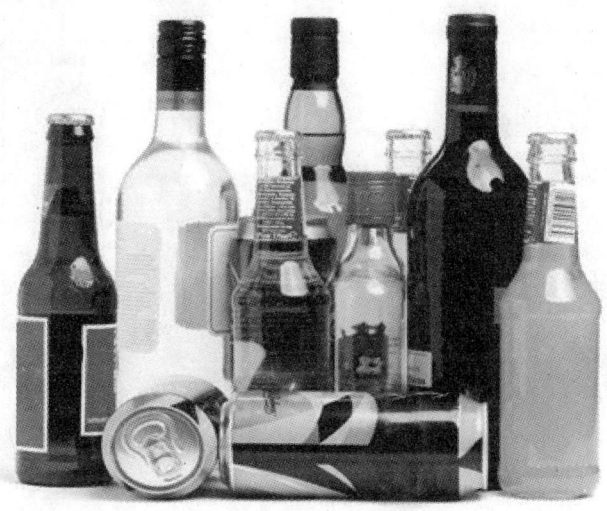

Some acne prone sufferers have indicated an immediate flare-up of the condition after the consumption of alcohol, more often after drinking beer or whiskey. In such circumstances, it is advisable to drastically decrease or abstain from alcohol if possible.

As alcohol is considered to be an astringent, some people believe that it can be applied topically on the skin over the acne spots or scars. But it may dry out the skin excessively, inflame it or make it itchy due to some allergic reaction without treating the underlying cause of the acne breakout.

Bacteria

Bacteria are unicellular micro-organisms present almost everywhere on earth–whether deep down in the oceans, seas, rivers or in the earth's crust, in the soil, in radioactive waste, in garbage and in almost any environment on the earth. Existing as both benign and virulent forms, bacteria can be present in all parts of the body.

The bacterium, *Propionibacterium acnes*, is present on the surface of the skin of all individuals. It remains benign in the skin but in certain individuals it causes the onset of acne more due to an unfavourable environment in the skin rather than by its own actions.

An oil based environment is ideal for *propionibacterium acnes* to thrive and multiply. When the sebaceous glands secrete excess oil or sebum, the number of this bacteria in the skin increases. When the pores of the skin are blocked, this bacterium thrives as it secretes chemicals that break down the pore walls and skin lesions are formed on the surface of the skin causing inflammation. As the exact mechanism of the bacteria in causing acne is still unclear, this is the probable role of the bacteria.

The bacteria can be treated using benzoyl peroxide, drugs from the tetracycline group and clove oil. However, the bacteria may become resistant to these drugs over a period of time.

Caffeine

Caffeine is a natural stimulant present in several foods, the main ones being cocoa and coffee. When we ingest small quantities of caffeine, there is a surge of adrenaline produced in the body. This leads to a fight or flight reaction. This is why many people believe that they cannot function without their morning cup of coffee. Sodas also contain high sources of caffeine and give teenagers the boost to get through the day despite late hours and less sleep. Many individuals who have less of the two R's—rest and recuperation resort to stimulants like coffee to help them get through the day. This does work for many and no long term effects are seen many a times. However, some people are highly allergic to this chemical compound called caffeine.

Some individuals, especially teenagers and even adults have reported an enhancement of their acne breakouts after the consumption of high caffeine based foods and drinks.

In this modern world with its own pressures, it is not possible to work long hours in stressful jobs without a few natural or artificial stimulants. It may be difficult but is always advisable for everyone to at least decrease their consumption of caffeine based products even if they cannot cut them out totally from their lives.

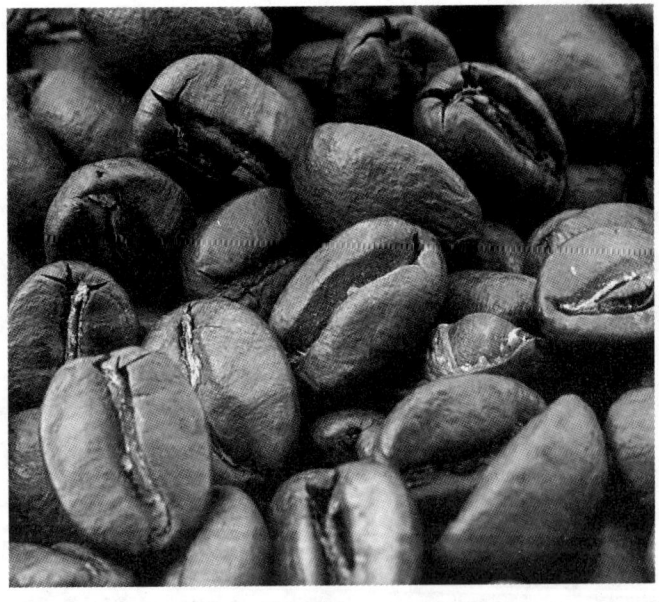

Cosmetics

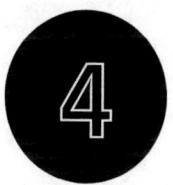

Cosmetics per se do not cause acne. However as with various other factors, they are capable of aggravating acne in sensitive individuals. **Acne cosmetica** as it is termed is generally seen as whiteheads and small bumps in various parts of the face including the hairline, below the eyes, the cheeks, etc. making it easier to identify the cosmetic culprit which may be a hair colour, eye make-up, foundation, moisturiser, etc.

It is a good idea to identify the product causing the skin to react and to stop using it. Oil based products generally have sebum derivatives which may aggravate the production of sebum in the skin. However, water based products may also react with the skin as they may have more synthetic chemicals which can act as toxins and further react with the skin. Non-comedogenic make-up is available. It is quite expensive and may or may not suit you individually.

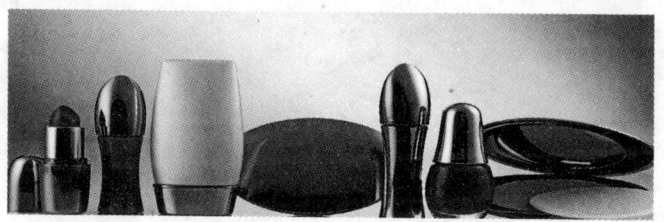

Dirt

A lot of research has been undertaken to prove that dirt does not cause acne. Yes, while this may be true, it is also true that a clean body like a clean mind harbours less diseases and conditions detrimental to humankind.

Washing one's face twice a day is something any individual can do and if an acne prone sufferer does so with a mild soap it can indeed benefit such individuals.

Dirt does not harm an acne prone individual directly, but indirectly it is always better to be clean and hygienic. Hence, a regular mild cleansing routine twice a day is beneficial for all.

Drugs

It is a well documented fact that certain drugs cause acne. However it is also absolutely essential that a person does not stop the usage of these drugs since they see breakouts of acne as a side effect of these drugs. Generally these categories of drugs are prescribed for much more serious and life threatening conditions that may be more important than an acne flare-up and it is advisable to contact a qualified dermatologist to find a solution to combat these side effects.

Some of the drugs which cause acne as a side effect in some individuals are as follows:

Anabolic Androgenic Steroids

Anabolic androgenic steroids, commonly known as anabolic steroids are drugs that are similar to the male sex hormone—testosterone. They increase body weight and muscular strength. Hence they are used and sometimes abused by many including male and female athletes and those who are keen on building muscles using short cuts. They have many potential side effects including the development of acne in both males and females.

DHEA or **Dehydroepiandrosterone** is an anabolic steroid available with a prescription in some countries. It is also available as an over the counter (OTC) drug in other countries. It is banned by the World Anti-doping Agency for athletes and is listed as a prohibited substance. It mimics the properties of androgenic hormones to some extent. It may cause acne in sensitive individuals.

It is generally recommended that people build their healthy bodies through a combination of proper diet and adequate exercise rather than resort to dietary supplements and anabolic steroids. A proper diet and exercise regime will not only make a person healthy but will also go a long way in decreasing their acne attacks.

Anticonvulsants

These drugs are a diverse group of medicines used to treat epileptic seizures and bipolar disorders. They prevent the frequency of convulsions and seizures and also act as mood stabilizers.

Some patients have reported an outbreak of acne due to the use of this class of drugs. This may be true in individual cases. However, other studies carried out have also shown that there is no link between these drugs and acne. It is recommended that such patients consult a registered dermatologist and treat their acne.

Barbiturates

These drugs act on the central nervous system. They are addictive by nature. They are mainly used to treat anxiety and epilepsy, and can be used as a general anaesthetic. They may cause acne outbreaks in some individuals. However, do not stop using them as they are often prescription drugs and it is better to consult a dermatologist if you find yourself developing any skin problems. Now-a-days, benzodiazepines are the class of drugs more commonly prescribed as these have fewer side effects.

Corticosteroids

Some synthetic corticosteroids are used to treat a diverse variety of ailments including asthma. They may cause acne outbreaks in sensitive individuals. Do not stop your medication if you find that you are developing acne as a side effect of these medications. Instead, consult a dermatologist and explore methods to decrease or diminish the outbreaks.

Lithium

Lithium is used to treat several mood disorders. It may also cause acne outbreaks in some individuals. Many studies have shown that lithium has a detrimental effect on skin causing acne, psoriasis and other skin ailments. The exact mechanism of how these conditions develop is still not known.

Do not stop taking lithium to stop the acne outbreaks. Perhaps your physician will decrease the amount of lithium prescribed if possible. Otherwise consult a dermatologist to find a method suitable to decrease the acne outbursts.

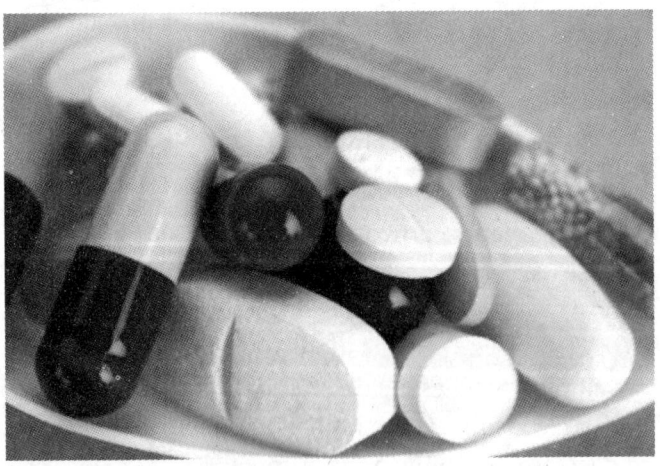

Artificial Sweetners

Artificial sweeteners are generally chemicals, both natural and synthetically manufactured. They may have had their structures altered to increase their sweetness when compared to sucrose or common sugar.

They are generally much cheaper than sugar and have much higher intensities of sweetness ranging from 30 times sweeter (cyclamate) to neotame which is 8000 times sweeter by weight. Thus, artificial sweeteners may be used in negligible quantities and hence do not increase the energy or calorific value of foods.

Artificial sweeteners may also cause acne. Almost all diet foods have artificial sweeteners. Many acne sufferers have complained that their acne flares up after consuming the so-called diet foods and drinks and we can surmise that the higher load of chemicals present in these processed foods may be aggravating the acne.

Baker's Yeast

Baker's yeast is generally used as a leavening agent while making breads and other bakery products. It is available as a liquid or in powder form. It is easily available in bakeries and supermarkets.

Baker's yeast may cause allergies in sensitive individuals. However, it is not considered as a common food allergen. It is an ingredient in most baked pastries and these baked products often cause acne flare-ups.

Some acne prone individuals have actually found that a small quantity of baker's yeast has helped to decrease their acne and even use small quantities (dissolved in water to make the yeast active) directly on their faces. This just goes to show that there is a lot of research to be done to find out the specific causes of acne and what may cause acne in one individual may treat the acne in another individual.

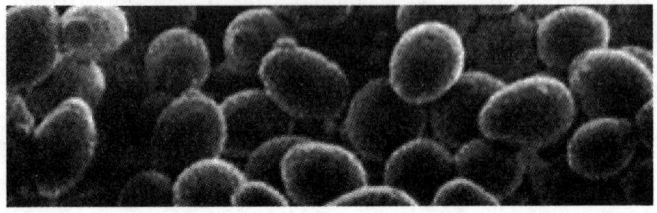

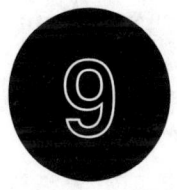 # Beef

Many kinds of meat including beef are said to cause acne in certain individuals. The cause of acne is attributed to the high fatty acid content of these foods. Saturated fats are unhealthy fats and even if they do not cause acne, eating them in limited quantities is beneficial for general health.

One theory proposed to substantiate the fact that beef causes acne is that digestion is slowed down by all types of meat and hence this leads to a build-up of different toxins in the body and some of these may get eliminated via the skin instead of the excretory system.

Others say that the use of growth hormone is permitted in some countries and this may be the cause of acne as the effect of hormones on acne is an acknowledged one.

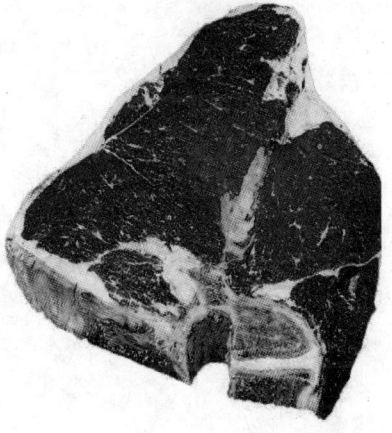

Check the effect of meat and meat products in your diet. If you cannot eliminate it totally from your diet, try to reduce the quantity you consume and see if you find any visible change in the parts of the body where your acne is the worst.

Broccoli

Iodine present naturally in foods is indeed a boon to humankind as it is an essential trace element required for the normal functioning of the body. Iodine deficiency in humans is indeed a worrying factor as it can lead to the development of cretinism which delays the normal development of infants and can also lead to mental retardation or the development of goitre in adults. Vegetables grown in iodine rich soil are generally considered as healthy and nutritious vegetables. Iodine is also supplemented in foods to promote general health and to help the thyroid gland to function normally.

However, acne prone individuals are sometimes susceptible to aggravation of symptoms after they consume foods rich in iodine including broccoli. Hence, broccoli may be considered as a potential acne aggravator in sensitive

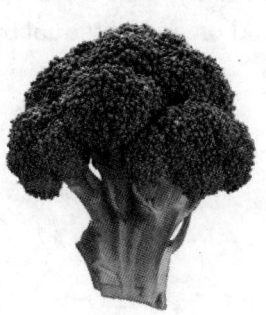

individuals. As yet, there is no specific research findings to substantiate or counter this claim.

There are also a group of acne sufferers who believe that the addition of broccoli to their diet has helped to improve their acne. As mentioned before, broccoli is a healthy and nutritious vegetable containing many essential micronutrients including selenium and some antioxidants and phytonutrients. Perhaps a combination of factors in broccoli and a nutritious diet that promotes good health may also be responsible for decreasing the incidence of acne in certain individuals.

If an acne prone individual notices an increase in inflammation or redness, it is better to avoid the consumption of broccoli. But do remember that all fruits and vegetables are protective foods so it is always good to include several servings of fruits and vegetables in the daily diet. Do avoid or include broccoli in your food on an individual basis.

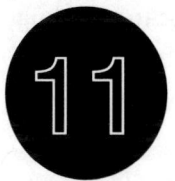

Candy

Candy covers a huge range of confectionary and sweets and is a food item that almost all of us eat more often than not. Generally, the major ingredient in most candies is sugar. Sugar has been considered as a culprit for causing acne by many as it definitely raises the glycemic index of foods. Foods with high glycemic index tend to increase the amount of glucose present in the blood stream and hence there is a greater secretion of insulin. After the consumption of foods with a high glycemic index, there is also an increased secretion of Insulin-like Growth Factor 1. This increased secretion of both insulin and IGF-1, increases the hormonal levels, especially those of testosterone. This in turn increases the production of sebum. As most of us know, an excess of sebum leads to blockage of pores in the skin and thus the final result is an outbreak of acne. However, there may also be another causative agent in the candy to which you may be allergic, like peanuts or artificial colours or flavours.

It is very difficult to cut out candy from the diet especially during adolescence but perhaps decreased consumption of sugar in the form of candies can help decrease the acne. If you find a specific type of candy causes more frequent or increasingly severe outbreaks of acne, avoid it.

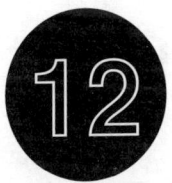 # Cheese

Since milk has been implicated in increasing the severity of acne, it follows that eating cheese can also increase the severity of acne.

Cheese has a lot of health benefits, being a good source of quality proteins and essential vitamins and minerals. But studies conducted on both cream cheese and cottage cheese shows that both of these cheeses increase the severity of acne.

It is advisable to try and find out whether cheese consumption has affected you individually before totally removing it from the diet. Generally, an elimination diet helps you to pinpoint allergens and other factors that affect the condition of your skin.

Some individuals feel that raw cheese (unpasteurised) obtained from organic milk may have more beneficial effects.

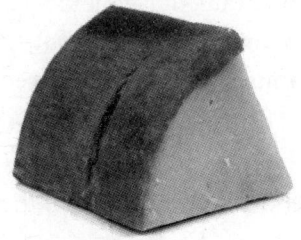

13. Chocolate

Most dermatologists believe that chocolates do not cause acne. However, many sufferers of acne confirm the fact that chocolate causes or aggravates their acne. Most people love chocolate and a very minuscule percentage of the population would like to identify chocolate as the culprit for the outbreak of their acne.

Perhaps it would be wise to make a note of the type of chocolate you are eating? Traditionally dark chocolate which has proportionately more of cocoa powder and less milk and sugar, is identified by most nutritionists, doctors and health care professionals as a food that is good for your general health. Two pieces of dark chocolate as a part of your daily diet has definitely proven to be a health benefit in several studies. Cocoa contains many protective phytochemicals which help maintain the general well being of the human body. Hence, it is important to note that dark chocolate in limited amounts is extremely good for you.

If you think your current out-burst of acne was due to consuming chocolate, do check the type of chocolate and the amount you have eaten and you will most probably find that either over-indulgence or very sugary and/or a milky chocolate were the causes.

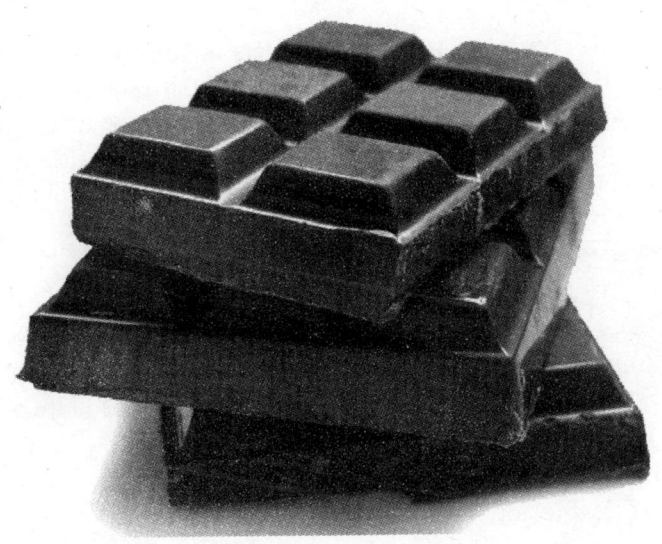

Corn

Studies on corn and corn products including corn on the cob, high fructose corn syrup and corn oil causing or aggravating acne, have implicated these products to a certain extent. Some people develop a mild allergy when they ingest corn products. Perhaps the allergic reaction further inflames acne already present in susceptible individuals.

High fructose corn syrup (HFCS) also has a high glycemic index and many studies have indicated that simple sugars play a major role in the incidence of acne. It is better to avoid processed foods with HFCS for general health as well as to avoid acne.

It may also be advisable for susceptible individuals to avoid corn starch. Corn starch may be used as an ingredient, both in foods and in cosmetics.

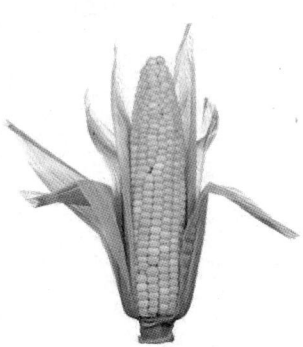

Cream

Since cream is derived from milk, it may also cause acne in many sensitive individuals. However, studies have proved that skimmed milk causes more frequent outbursts of acne rather than whole milk. Hence, cream may cause mild symptoms of acne when compared to skimmed milk. As with other foods which may or may not cause allergic reactions in individuals, it is better to check out the long term effects of eliminating cream from the diet.

Eggs

Eggs are an excellent source of complete proteins. They contain all the essential amino acids required for optimum growth. During childhood and adolescence, making egg a part of the diet definitely identifies with a healthy diet.

Eggs are also well proven to be allergens. Some individuals have allergic reactions to eggs. It is said that the smell itself might trigger the allergy. However, some feel that the egg yolk does more harm and they can consume the white of the egg safely.

If you suffer from acne, perhaps you could go slow on your intake of eggs. While an egg a day may be ideal for most adolescents, if you believe it increases your acne or is responsible for it, do avoid its consumption. Check out if the entire egg or just the yolk causes your allergy. Also cook the egg using different cooking methods like frying, baking and boiling and then eliminate the type of cooking method that aggravates your acne outbreak. Generally eggs are a healthy and tasty food and unless you find them specifically affecting you, there is no need to eliminate them from the adolescent diet.

Causes of Acne | 53

Egg white as a face mask has been used for ages. It is said that the egg white naturally tightens the pores of the skin. Use it to improve the texture of your skin if it suits you. Others recommend the use of the yolk or even the whole egg. Always do a small 'patch' test and try the effect of the egg on a small part of the skin and then use it confidently. Remember not to keep the mask on for too long. Just keep it till there is a tight feeling on the face and then wash it using clean water and see if you feel a visible difference. If you do feel a difference continue using it, if not stop using it.

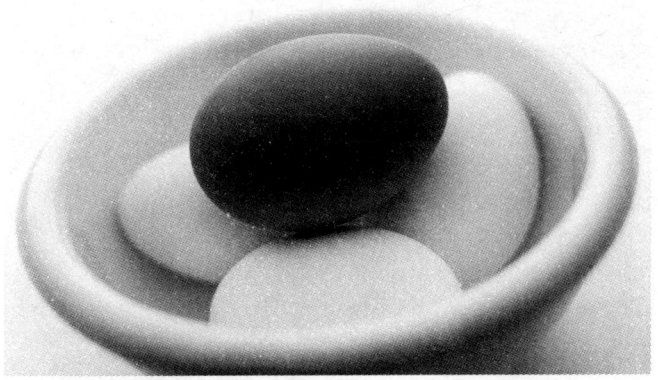

Garlic

The potential use of garlic as an antiviral or antibiotic has been documented in various alternative schools of medicine. Mainstream or the western systems of medicine are not really inclined towards research on natural alternatives to health.

However some people are allergic to garlic. As with almost any natural food, individuals are susceptible to allergies. Sometimes the natural food itself may not be the cause but a potential allergen associated with harvest, post-harvest, during processing or post-processing may be responsible for the allergic reaction.

If you use garlic, either crushed or as a juice or in combination with vinegar or any other substance, do go slow as all natural compounds in their raw form have enzymes which may just aggravate sensitive skin.

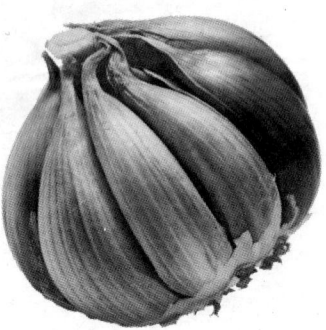

Gluten

Wheat, barley, rye and oats contain proteins in the form of gluten. Gluten has been a potential allergen for a cross section of the population worldwide. In fact, there is a thriving food industry which makes a lot of gluten free products (and a lot of money too) for sufferers of this allergen.

A person allergic to gluten may find that it creates problems both in the digestive system and on the skin. Inflammation of the skin may be a common reaction when sensitive individuals eat gluten based foods. Individuals, who are sensitive to gluten, may find their acne is exacerbated when they consume gluten based products.

It is indeed a good idea for acne prone individuals to check their diets for potential allergens and avoid foods which may further aggravate their condition. Don't let gluten intolerance become the reason for your acne to become more severe.

There is no strong evidence supporting the theory that a gluten free diet may stop or decrease acne. However, there is reason to believe that a large number of individuals have seen skin benefits after they have been advised to go on a gluten-free diet. It is not easy to follow a gluten free diet and it is better to go on such a diet after allergy tests have proven that you have a high level of gluten intolerance or if you have tried all other potential allergens and other probable causes of acne. If other causes do not exist you may need to eliminate gluten as a final probable cause of aggravating your acne either by realizing it yourself through trial and error or by undergoing tests designed to identify allergens.

Ice cream

Ice cream is a delicious food and can be eaten by most of us at any time of the day or night. Unfortunately though, it may not be a recommended food for some of you who suffer from acne.

The main ingredients of ice cream include dairy and sugar. As per research studies, both dairy and sugar have been implicated as ingredients that aggravate acne. Some researchers have concluded that there is an association between acne and the consumption of milk. Further research may prove that they also may be causative factors.

Many individuals have agreed to the fact that their acne has improved after they decreased or eliminated ice cream from their daily diet. Low dairy or no dairy ice creams with low sugar may be alternatives. However, do not forget the fact that for general health, all foods, especially the non-healthy ones should be eaten in limited quantities.

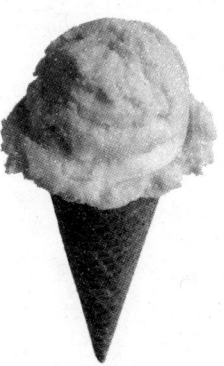

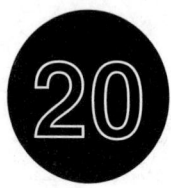

Lamb

Lamb, like other meats, has been considered as a food that promotes the development of acne in teenagers. Lamb, as a red meat, is high in saturated fatty acids and these saturated fats can increase the production of sebum in the body.

Currently, many studies are being carried out on the correlation of diet rich in fatty acids in relation to the incidence of acne. As with many other foods, it is advisable to eat limited quantities of lamb and if it aggravates your acne, it is better to reduce consumption or if possible, completely eliminate lamb from your diet.

Mangoes

Mango is a delicious fruit. It is a rich source of many nutrients including protective phytochemicals and other vital nutrients. It has a delicious taste and appealing colour that tends to stimulate our senses. Mangoes are also a fair source of dietary fibre and carbohydrates. They are low in proteins and fat. They contain appreciable quantities of vitamins including beta carotene, which is converted to vitamin A in the body. Beta carotene is a protective phytochemical which mops up free radicals which are naturally produced in the body and are harmful. Mangoes

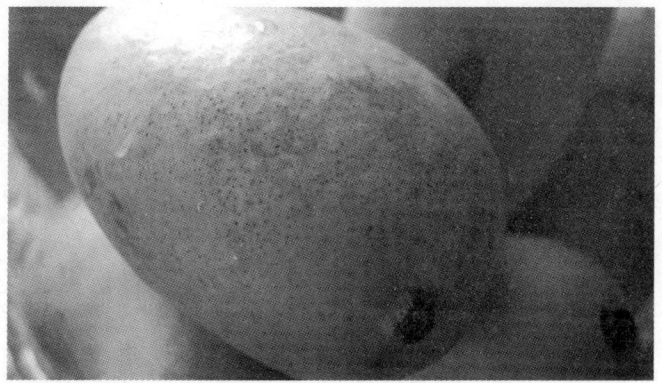

also contain vitamin B and many essential minerals including iron.

On the whole, mangoes are good for health. No major studies have implicated mangoes as a cause of acne. There is no direct corroboration between mangoes and acne. Nevertheless, the mango peel may cause an allergic reaction in some individuals. This may lead to skin infections and finally bacterial infection which are common causes of acne.

Another factor responsible for the outbreak of acne, probably due to mangoes may be the over-consumption of the fruit. Any acne prone individual may not see an increase in the condition unless they consume large amounts of foods. A food has to be consumed in optimum quantities and over-indulgence in any food generally has medical consequences.

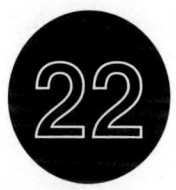

Margarine

The term margarine is used to describe a wide range of products used to substitute butter. Today there is a wide range of margarines produced by a large number of manufacturers.

Margarines generally contain trans fats which are harmful for the body as they block or clog arteries supplying oxygenated blood from the heart to various organs. As technology progresses, many margarine manufacturers have lowered or eliminated the amount of trans fat in their products.

However, a few additives are still added in the manufacture of margarine. These additives have been implicated in causing or aggravating acne in sensitive individuals. There are not many specific studies on the effect of margarine on acne prone individuals. However, it 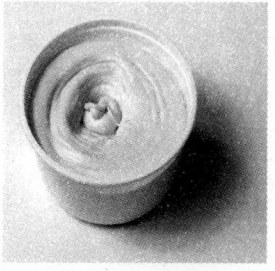 is wise to avoid margarine if you see yourself breaking out with acne after consuming it.

Milk

Milk is a healthy food for most people except those who have been diagnosed as suffering from lactose intolerance. Such individuals are unable to digest lactose—the sugar naturally present in milk. However, some studies have shown that milk can also lead to an increase in acne in adolescents as the hormones present in milk may stimulate the production of acne.

Studies conducted on adolescents in 2005 did implicate milk as a causative factor of acne. Thus, care should be taken to ensure that there is a sufficient intake of calcium from other sources if milk is eliminated from the teenage diet.

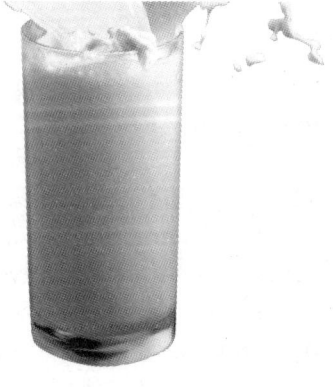

Although there aren't any studies on adults, some adults have reported improvement in the incidence of acne after they cut down their consumption of milk. Research studies prove that skimmed milk seems to cause more acne than whole milk.

Though there is no definite proof that drinking milk causes acne, some studies have shown that milk consumption aggravates the severity of acne and a milk-free diet does not eliminate but may decrease the severity of acne in some, but not all individuals

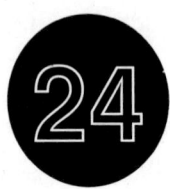

Mushroom

Mushrooms are extremely important fungi that have a lot of health benefits in the form of proteins, vitamins and minerals. They are an important source of vital nutrients in a vegetarian diet. However, as with other foods it is possible that they may cause allergic reactions or exacerbate acne in sensitive individuals.

Being a fungus, though a healthy one, may be the reason why mushrooms affect certain individuals. However, there is a wide variety of mushrooms

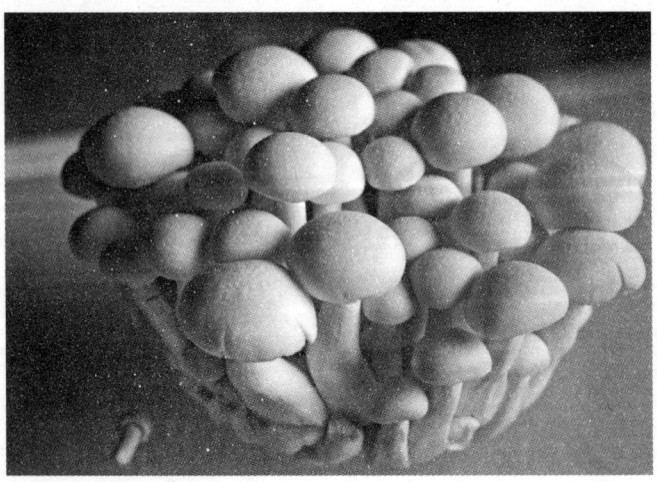

available and there is no need to eliminate them from your diet unless you are totally sure that it has been the cause of your breakout.

Healthy food is a must for all individuals. Yes, it is possible that some foods have natural allergens and affect a miniscule amount of the human population. But this does not mean that one avoids all potentially allergic foods unless one has personally seen the allergic effects.

If you suspect mushrooms to be the cause of your acne, avoid them. If not, go ahead and consume these delicious fungi nature has provided for humankind.

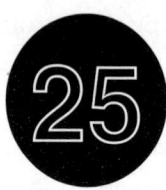# Oysters

Considered as an aphrodisiac by many, oysters are a part of the shellfish family which includes shrimps, clams, mussels and scallops. This group of sea creatures has often been implicated as common food allergens. If you are allergic to these foods, there is a great possibility that you may find your outbreaks of acne increasing in intensity and aggravation as allergens generally affect the skin and increase inflammation.

However if you find that you do not develop any allergies after eating shellfish, go ahead and enjoy these

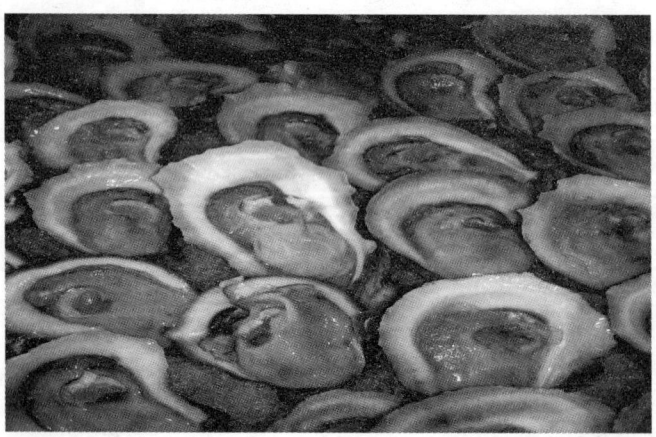

delicacies which not only taste delicious but are also a good source of many essential micronutrients including zinc, some proteins, vitamins including vitamin B_{12}, but remember that they also contain cholesterol.

Unless you are specifically allergic to shellfish, this group of food will not cause or aggravate your acne breakouts.

Peanuts

Peanuts, otherwise known as monkey nuts, groundnuts, etc., across different cultures are among the most popular natural known foods and a universally favourite snack, spread or oil. Roasted or boiled peanuts are a common snack that transcend all barriers of age, culture, status and ethnicity. Peanut butter is popular across all age groups and peanut/groundnut oil is an excellent source of essential unsaturated fatty acids.

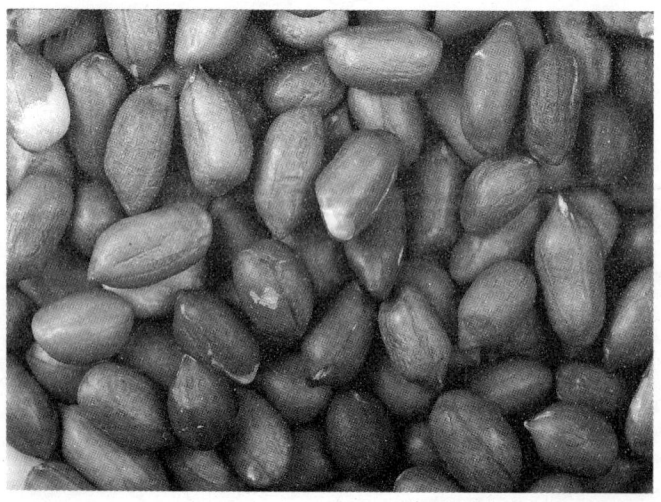

Peanuts, eaten in moderate quantities, supply protein, essential fatty acids, vitamins and minerals which are essential for normal well being. It is important to note that the key word is moderation as a high fat intake, even if it comprises mainly of essential fatty acids is never recommended as a part of a balanced diet.

However, this delicious and wonderful food is one of the most common allergens among a certain percentage of individuals worldwide. Even traces of peanut in processed foods may lead to intensive allergic reactions in sensitive individuals.

Eczema is a common symptom amongst many that manifests itself on the skin of these individuals and untreated eczema may also lead to the development of acne in these individuals. Acne may be a secondary reaction rather than a primary reaction to the ingestion of peanuts.

Peanuts are an excellent and healthy snack but if you think it may affect your acne, avoid it. If not, enjoy this delicious nut which is a bounty from nature's warehouse.

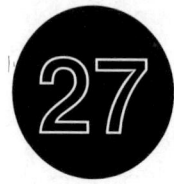

Pickles

There is absolutely no proof to link pickles with the outbreak of acne. However, many individuals who consume pickles feel that there is an increase in acne within a brief period of time after consumption.

Pickles per se may not cause acne, but care has to be taken not to consume pickles in large quantities.

Using a small quantity of pickle may not only improve the taste of your meal but may also stimulate the digestive juices in the body and improve digestion. Hygienically prepared pickles using natural ingredients may actually have beneficial effects when consumed in very minimal quantities.

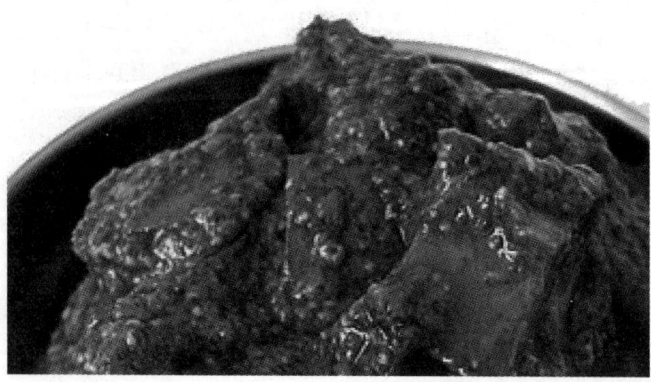

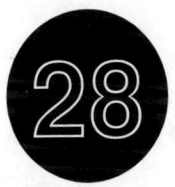

Pineapple

Some people suffer from allergic reactions to acidic fruits including pineapple. Some people feel a slight burning sensation on their tongues due to the astringent nature of the fruit. If this is the case, it is better to avoid pineapples, if you are both allergic and have an acne prone skin.

However, if you notice no allergic reactions, pineapples are indeed good for acne prone skin. No specific study has been conducted on the effects of pineapple on acne prone skin but it has been reported that many users find their skins clear up when they eat pineapple. Raw fruits generally have a good effect on decreasing or diminishing acne scars. In fact, crushed pineapple pulp is used on the face. When the pulp is used for a short period of time, it has actually lightened acne scars.

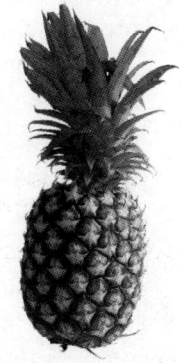

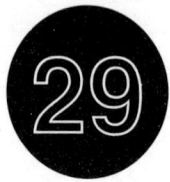

Potatoes

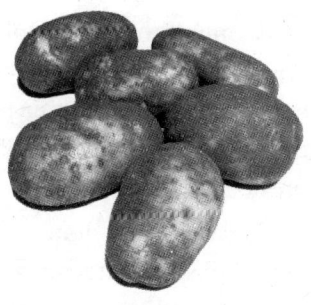

Potatoes are a healthy vegetable containing carbohydrate, some protein, a fair amount of vitamin C and other vitamins and minerals. They are best consumed by boiling or steaming. Jacket potatoes (baked) are also fairly nutritious though some amounts of vitamins are lost while baking. Stir fried potatoes are a much better way of consuming potatoes than frying them, but that's how most of the world consumes potatoes–as chips. Potato chips contain enough fat to negate the positive influence of this tasty and easily available source of nutrients. Fried foods are detrimental to acne and hence, a large or even a medium bag of chips may just aggravate your acne further.

Raw potato, rubbed in the form of slices gently on the face or scrapped potato as a crushed pulp on the face is known to lighten acne scars. Do not keep the potato on for too long as it will dry the skin.

Refined Wheat Flour

Refined wheat flour is used as an ingredient to make many products including white bread, most cakes and pastries. It is less nutritious than whole wheat flour as most of the vitamins naturally present in whole wheat are lost during milling. It is often bleached to make it white and the chemicals used to bleach the flour may cause allergic adverse reactions in individuals. On the whole, it has smaller amounts of essential nutrients when compared with whole wheat flour and has a higher glycemic index.

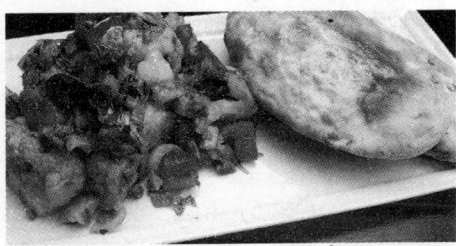

Refined wheat flour is not recommended in normal diets. Hence it is better if acne prone adolescents cut out or drastically reduce their intake of refined wheat flour.

Rice

The theory that rice causes acne is almost totally unsubstantiated. Eating either white rice or brown rice in moderate quantities is an integral part of the diet. Rice is an essential part of many Asian diets and there has been no massive incidence of acne outbreak due to the consumption of rice.

Since white rice is refined and highly polished, the glycemic index increases and it is digested much faster than unmilled rice. Hence, large quantities may increase but not cause acne. It is important to note that brown rice or unmilled rice is higher in nutrients and also has a lower glycemic index when compared to white rice.

Consuming food with a low glycemic index is definitely beneficial for general health and for sufferers of acne too. It is not necessary to stop eating rice even if it is white rice but it is advisable to eat it in moderate amounts.

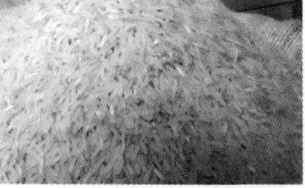

Ready Meals

In today's fast paced world, 'ready meals' are an extremely convenient option as food for all people, from the harassed and over-worked office goer to the stay-at-home homemaker who uses these meals for convenience.

However these meals, despite the convenience they offer, are more often than not laden with empty calories or flavor enhancers. They have a long list of additives and preservatives which many consumers do not even bother to read.

It is generally advisable for a normal person to eat such meals more on a convenience basis rather than as a part of their routine food habits. It is even more essential for an acne prone individual to avoid these meals almost absolutely, unless perhaps it is the only food available.

There is no research available to show that these meals affect acne but they have the highest potential to trigger acne among most individuals. They contain larger amounts of artificial ingredients and these additives and preservatives are more likely to cause allergic reactions in individuals. Since there is not a single clear factor which is implicated as the cause of acne, it is possible that acne could be a result of food allergies and hence it is a good idea to avoid potential allergens.

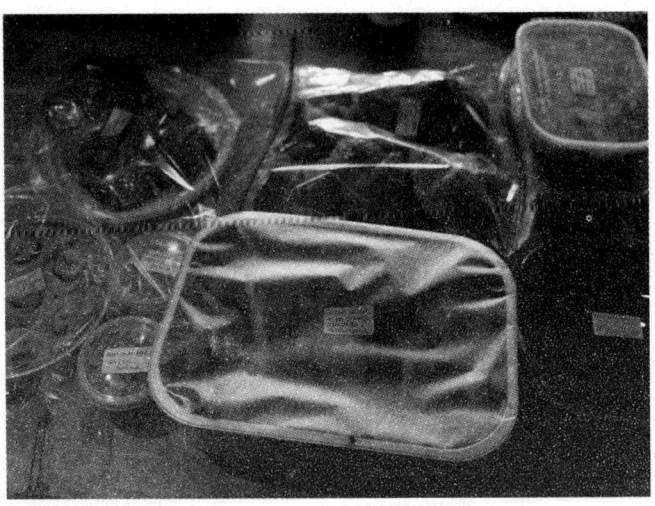

Sesame

Sesame oil obtained from sesame seeds is also known as **gingelly oil**. Sesame, as seeds or oil is used as an ingredient in various cuisines. It has an ancient history and has been used as an ingredient and spice in several cultures. It has a distinctive taste. Although sesame seeds are found in various colours, black sesame seeds are considered to be the healthiest amongst all. It is rich in nutrients and contains several vitamins and essential minerals and antioxidants.

The oil is generally used to soften dry skin and as a nourishment for the skin. It may be combined with turmeric powder or used by itself.

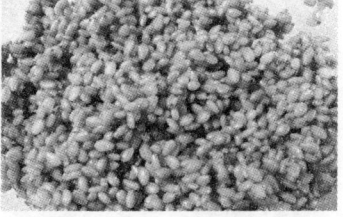

Some individuals have reported that their acne has increased after the application of sesame oil to their skin. Please avoid using it if it increases your acne.

 Soy or Soya Milk

Soya milk is a nutritious food. It has good quality proteins, vitamins of the B complex group, isoflavones and minerals. It is often used as a substitute for milk when a person is lactose intolerant.

Soy or soya milk is frequently consumed in the Far East and many parts of South-east Asia including China, Japan, Korea, Singapore and Malaysia. Recently, other parts of the world have also begun consuming soya milk or using it as a substitute for milk with cereals,

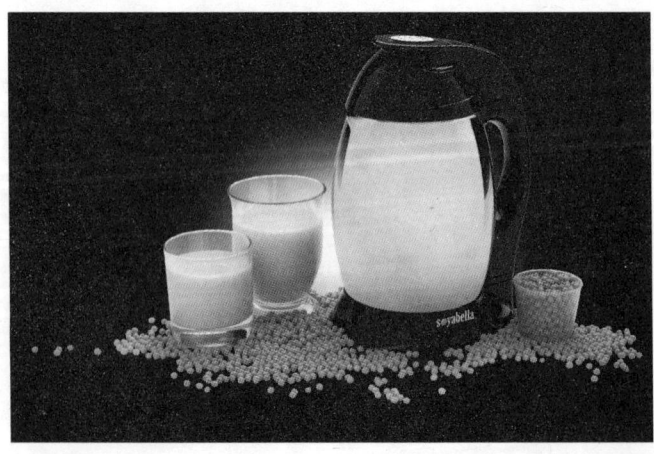

health drinks, etc. Many acne prone individuals have tried to replace milk with soya milk. Some have had some success while others have found out that their acne outbursts have increased in severity.

Japan uses a lot of soya milk and the incidence of acne is low in the country. Thus, it may not be possible to implicate soy as a causative agent of acne. Research studies have to be carried out and then a conclusion may be drawn.

On the other hand, soya milk may be a potential allergen and many individuals who replaced milk with soya milk may have had individual allergic reactions to the product. As with other foods, it is preferable to check whether one has allergies through tests or through eliminating the probable allergen from one's diet.

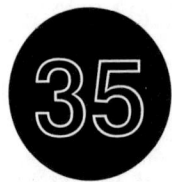

Spelt

Spelt is a species of wheat with a complex history. It is a hybrid which may have developed around fifth BC and is now mainly cultivated in parts of Europe. It is a nutritious food with carbohydrates, proteins, a small amount of fat and various vitamins and minerals. Spelt is used both as a whole grain and as spelt flour. The flour may be used to make bread, biscuits and other bakery products. It is also used to make pastas. It contains gluten.

Individuals who are prone to food allergies resulting from sensitivity to gluten or wheat and its products are also advised to avoid spelt and its products. It may trigger inflammation and exacerbate the acne formed in sensitive individuals.

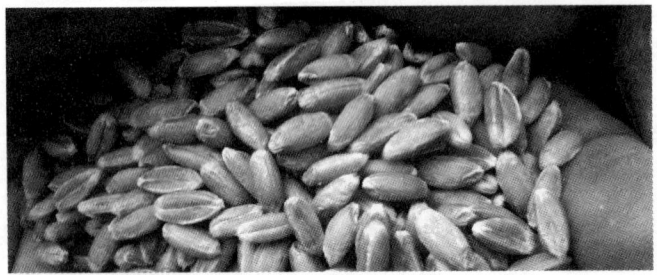

Spicy Food

Spicy food, is to some extent an ubiquitous part of the Indian and many Asian palates. The thought of eating bland food day-in and day-out to decrease or avoid acne may not be an easy step for lovers of spice. In fact, a certain amount of spice in life, both literally and emotionally is essential. Many spices have desirable qualities and help in digesting foods. Our Asian ancestors have documented the uses of these spices much before modern research had indeed proved their

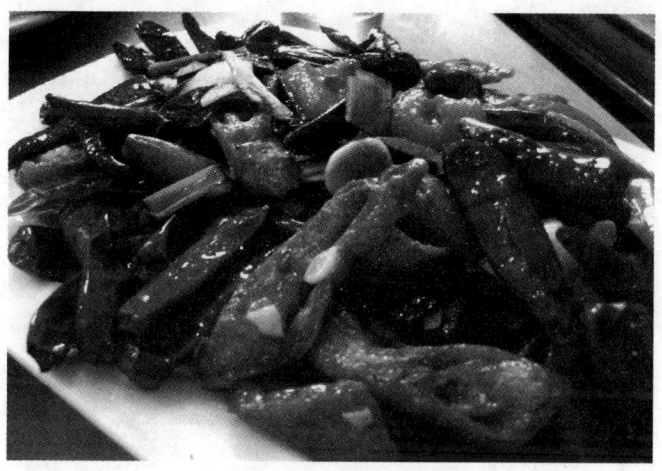

healing properties. **Capsaicin**, the active component in various types of chillies is used to relive aches and pains, as well as strains and sprains. **Curcumin** obtained from turmeric is used to treat various conditions including several cancers, arthritis and Alzheimer's disease. Other spices have been proven to have many curative properties as well though not as much through western research as Indian and Asian systems of medicine.

All spices have beneficial value when consumed in moderation. If an acne prone individual see an immediate flare-up, perhaps s(he) may avoid consuming large quantities of spicy foods and decrease the amount of oil used along with the spices. It is not necessary to avoid total consumption of spices when you are used to them as this will decrease the satiety value of foods.

Sugars

Life without natural and artificial sweetness is not something anyone living in the modern world can contemplate. Through the ages, humankind has developed a sweet tooth whether it is for the natural sugars present in many fruits, a few vegetables and honey, or artificial low calorie equivalents. The refining of sugar from cane or beet has been a major processing breakthrough but has also lead to a world where there is more of an emphasis on processed rather than natural foods.

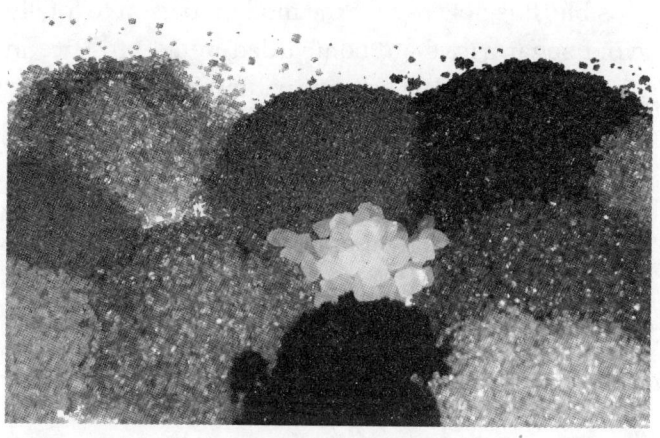

Sugar may be consumed in small quantities and preferably from natural sources for our body to function optimally. Sugar gives us a very pleasurable feeling and sensation. Hence, we crave for it in so many foods and consume it in excess. Complex sugars, which break down more slowly in the body don't taste as good as simple sugars but are much healthier.

Excess sugar in the diet leads to obesity. Improper metabolism of sugars in the body leads to diabetes. Sugar has been implicated as a cause of acne in various studies conducted as it affects the production of IGF-1, an insulin-like growth factor that affects the normal functioning of the skin.

It is always advisable to consume complex rather than simple sugars in their natural form as much as possible. It is not easy for the modern person to totally avoid sugar as we are bombarded by its presence in various products, but using its natural form is definitely advisable. If you cannot avoid it, at least decrease your consumption of modern sugars and you may see an improvement in the severity of your acne outbreaks as well as an improvement in general health.

Tuna

Tuna is a healthy food as it is an excellent source of omega-3 fatty acids, good quality proteins and several vitamins and minerals. It is generally recommended as a part of a healthy diet. It has a high content of iodine. However, high iodine content has also been considered as a causative factor that aggravates acne. No conclusive studies have been made so far. If you think you may have observed your acne flaring up after having tuna, perhaps you should avoid it. Sometimes tuna, is found to be contaminated with high levels of mercury. Mercury is a toxic heavy metal and can disrupt the normal functioning of your body.

Otherwise it is a safe and healthy food that can form a major part of your diet.

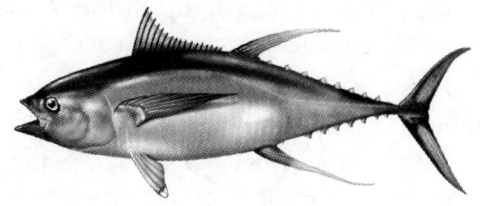

Trans Fats

Essential fatty acids, as the name suggests are essential for the normal functioning of the human body. Fat obtained from monounsaturated and polyunsaturated sources (obtained mainly from plant sources) are generally considered as sources of good fat whereas saturated fatty acids which form a part of most animal foods are not as healthy. However, many vegetable oils are hydrogenated (hydrogen is added as the oil is processed) to give a smooth feel and longer shelf life, especially to fried foods. This hydrogenated fat or trans fat is not broken down in the body and may even compete with the good fat present in the body leading to several problems. It also has adverse effects on various organs in the body including the heart and liver. It causes obesity which in turn is linked to the causative factor of many other chronic diseases. This fat also clogs skin pores leading to the formation of acne.

Trans fat is absolutely unessential for the normal functioning of the human body. It does not contain any essential fatty acids. A normal human being doesn't need to make it a part of their daily diet. So it is very important that an acne sufferer tries to cut out trans fats totally from their diet. It is essential to read labels as it is mandatory to mention the amount of trans fat present in all processed foods.

Many acne prone individuals have noticed that their acne disappear or decrease after they eliminate trans fats from their daily meals.

 # Walnut

Any nutritionist will tell you that all nuts are good for health. They contain essential fatty acids. They contain protein. They contain vitamins and minerals so it is indeed strange to read that such a healthy food may cause acne.

Some individuals have found that their acne flares up when they eat walnuts. There may be two reasons for this–the first one being that walnuts contain more of omega-6 fatty acids when compared to omega-3 fatty acids and the ratio between these fatty acids is important. If the diet already contains sufficient omega-6 fatty acids and the amount of these acids

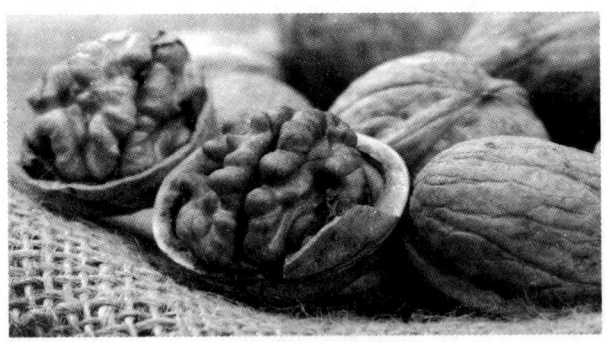

increases due to the consumption of walnuts the result could be an acne breakout.

Another reason could be that too many nuts are being consumed. Most people will agree that it is difficult to stop eating nuts. They are called healthy foods, they taste delicious and they are easy to carry or obtain.

So if you find your acne breaks out after eating walnuts, eliminate them from your diet initially. Then you may try to introduce small quantities and see if they affect your skin. If they do, avoid them totally. If they don't, continue enjoying these delicious and nutritious nuts.

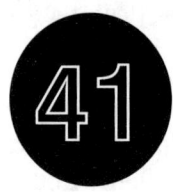 # Wheat Bran

The outer shell of the wheat grain, the wheat bran, is a good source of fibre. It also contains some protein, minimal amounts of fat, some good quality vitamin B, magnesium and trace amounts of iron. It is nutritious and is added to baked goods to improve their nutritional quality. However, as with other wheat products, some individuals who are allergic to wheat and gluten must avoid using wheat bran.

Although there are no specific studies correlating the use of wheat bran with acne, it better to avoid its consumption especially if you see the intensity of your

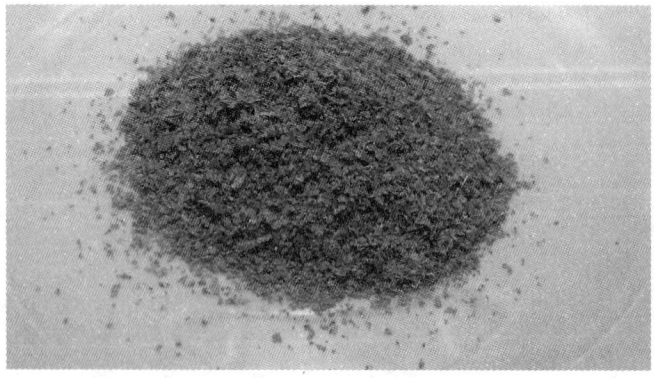

outbreaks increasing after eating any wheat based product.

If you have found that individually you have no adverse reaction to wheat and wheat products, please consume wheat bran in limited quantities. It may also be used as a face mask with honey and has cleared the skin of some individuals.

Wheat Germ

The embryo of the wheat kernel is called **wheat germ**. It is a rich source of nutrients and contains polyunsaturated fatty acids, proteins, some fibre, vitamins from the B complex group, vitamin E and also small quantities of iron. If you find that it suits your skin, it is advisable to supplement your diet with small amounts of wheat germ as it is good for general health

However, as with other wheat based products, if you are allergic to it, it is advisable to avoid wheat germ as it may trigger inflammation and extreme sensitivity in the skin of certain individuals.

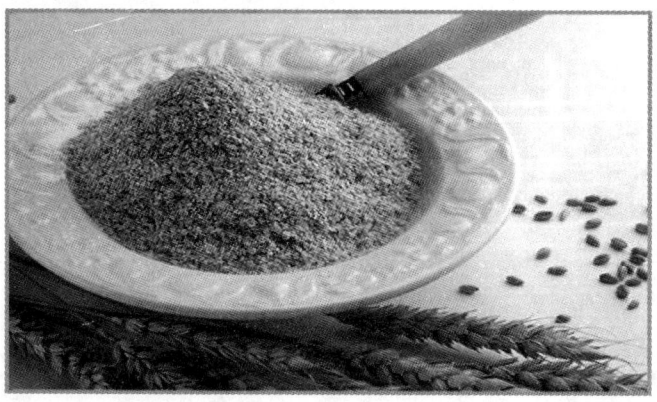

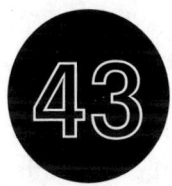

Wheat Flour

Wheat and wheat products such as wheat flour have been implicated as foods that cause acne. Many foods including pasta, breakfast cereals, a variety of breads, pastries, nutrition bars, etc. contain whole wheat or wheat flour. It is advisable to read the labels, as all processed foods have to list the ingredients present. Now-a-days, it is also possible to see the list of ingredients present in the menus in some restaurants.

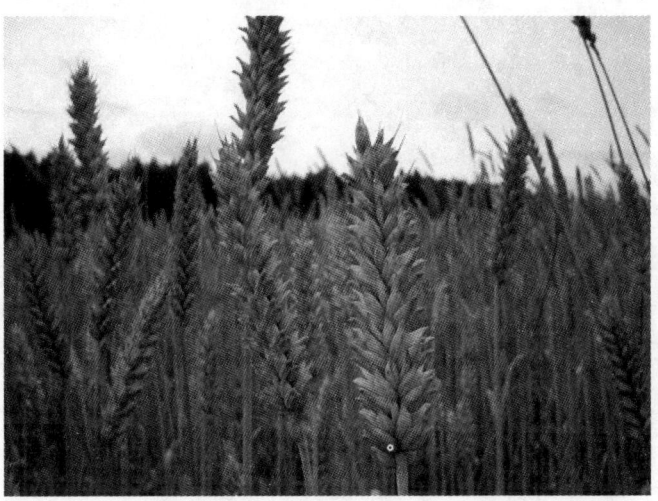

The exact mechanism is unknown but a few theories on how wheat causes acne have been floated around. However, none of these theories have been substantiated. Some theorists say that wheat and its products raise the glycemic index and hyperglycemia may cause the acne to flare-up. Others say that gluten, the protein present in wheat, is the major cause while others may be genetically prone to react adversely to wheat and its products.

Elimination diet is the best method of testing whether you are allergic to wheat and wheat products.

Genetics

Unfortunately for humankind, genetics is not kind to families. Acne occurs through generations and infants and children of acne sufferers also have a tendency to produce increased amounts of sebum naturally. Acne occurs predominantly in families which have a history of the condition. It affects both the males and females, and even twins. Clinical studies have proven that there is a strong link of acne occurring in families through generations. A few studies, to determine the genetic base for acne in generations, have been conducted. Studies on twins have shown that there is strong evidence that genetics plays a major role in

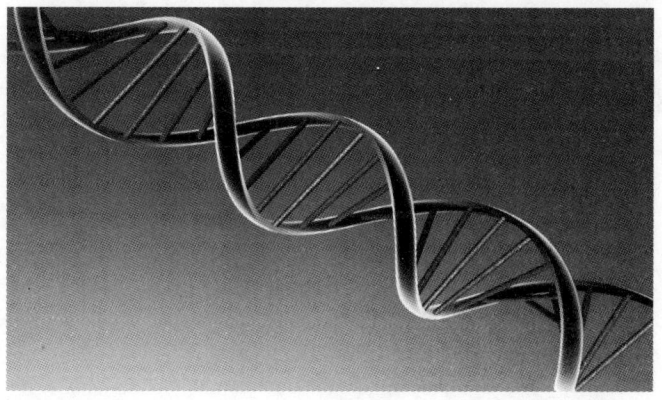

the formation of acne. Other studies on infants and neonatals have also shown that hereditary factors contribute to higher sebum levels.

More studies have shown that people with a history of acne running in the family find that they have earlier occurrences of acnes, more therapeutic difficulties and increased number of acne lesions.

However, as research is progressing, humankind has more and more opportunities to deal with and find cures for acne. Thus, despite the fact that one may have a predisposition towards acne, there is hope, as dermatologists are constantly researching on the subject. Acne is a common condition in many parts of the world and is present almost uniformly and commonly during adolescence in different cultures.

Hormones

A relationship between the onset of acne and hormones has been well established since decades. Acne generally occur in teens during pre-puberty and at the onset of puberty in both males and females. Adult acne is mainly confined to females though males have also shown to have outbreaks. Most women suffer from acne flare-ups just before their menstrual cycles, during pregnancy, pre-menopause and at the onset of menopause.

Generally the male hormones or androgenic hormones including testosterone and dihydrotestosterone are the hormones implicated as causative factors. Oestrogen and progestin have also been found to cause acne. However, recent research has shown that prostaglandins may also be one of the causative factors for the onset of pre-menstrual acne due to their vasoactive properties. Women suffering from PCOS (polycystic ovary syndrome) seem to be extra susceptible to suffering from acne attacks. Research indicates that women who have PCOS have elevated levels of androgen.

Studies on adult women with acne symptoms have shown that suppressing androgen has helped to reduce and treat acne breakouts in many women.

Other hormones including insulin and IGF1 have also shown to be involved in the incidence of acne in individuals.

To maintain a hormonal balance in the body, it is essential to consult an endocrinologist. Despite the various oral therapy medicines including birth control pills available for severe and chronic cases of acne it is better to consult specialists. It is also prudent to note that some of the treatments prescribed have side effects, may have detrimental effects and need constant supervision. Balancing a healthy lifestyle with sufficient exercise and a stress free life may go a long way in preventing major flare-ups. Medication for acne is an option when side effects from prescriptions are minimal and should be undertaken with regular medical supervision.

# Occupation

Can one's occupation increase outbreaks of acne? Yes, but in today's modern world there are many precautions one can take to prevent acne breakouts and this acne is distinct from the more common types seen in most individuals and can be treated.

Some people feel that working in hot and humid kitchens for long hours increases the breakout of acne in sensitive individuals. There is a condition called tropical acne where it is believed that hot and humid weather aggravates the formation of acne. Dry heat is comparatively safer. Others say that working in factories and industries, and being exposed to tars, organic solvents, petroleum products, chlorine based processes and other chemicals may worsen acne.

Studies on workers who were exposed to dust and vapours of solvents used in the coal tar industry showed that they developed a variety of skin related conditions including acne. Some amount of prevention of acne outbreaks was achieved by using protective gear, changing clothes frequently and maintaining high levels of hygiene with washing up and showering after immediate exposure to these chemicals. Workers exposed to halogenated aromatics mainly chlorine, iodides and bromides may develop a condition called **chloracne** which develops after direct exposure or inhalation or accidental ingestion of the halogens. In these cases it is essential to treat acne at the earliest as it may lead to future complications.

Acne prone individuals can take precautions to minimize all aggravating causes of acne and need not take drastic steps as changing their occupation to prevent acne. However, high levels of personal hygiene, minimal direct exposure to detrimental chemicals and cleanliness of both body and attire go a long way in the prevention of occupational acne.

Pressure

Sometimes it is very difficult to diagnose the cause of acne. A rare individual might find that he or she is unable to cure mild bouts of acne despite trying many medications and following a balanced and healthy lifestyle.

This is when it is time to explore uncommon factors and lesser researched causes like pressure on the skin due to the use of helmets, chin straps, tight collars and even suspenders. These are fairly unlikely causes for acne among most individuals. However it is better to rule out these causes and lead an as much as possible acne-free life.

Smoking

'Smoking is injurious to health'–it is a warning most of us have seen throughout our lives. 'Smoking causes cancer' is another common warning many of us are aware of. But do many of us know that cigarette or allied products let out innumerable carcinogens some of whose documented effects are not as yet known?

There is a lot of contradictory research on the effect of smoking on the incidence of acne flare-ups. Some studies find a direct correlation while others do not. Studies conducted by some scientists have concluded that smoking is a factor that contributes to both the prevalence and the severity of acne.

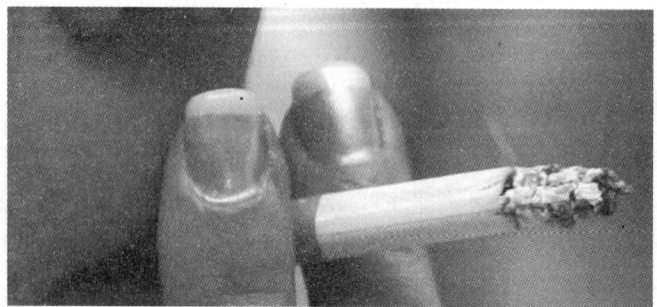

Just because a direct correlation is not found, one should not discount the harmful effects of smoking. There are so many unknown compounds yet to be studied and hence there is a wide probability that these indirectly, if not directly cause acne. However, studies have found a direct link between smoking and adult acne (non-inflammatory acne) in women. So if you have had acne as a youth and smoke, the chance of your acne clearing up naturally with a balanced lifestyle or with the help of dermatologists will decrease. Your acne may follow you in your adult years in its non-inflammatory form.

Many individuals report that their acne has cleared up after they quit smoking. Some have also seen an immediate outbreak after quitting but that may be the body's way of detoxification as these flare-ups start clearing away naturally when a healthy regime is followed.

Many acne cures take a while and instant results are noticed in some but not all individuals as they change their routine habits to healthy ones whether it is eating a balanced diet, or exercising or having a regular cleansing routine, or decreasing stress, or following an endocrinologist's advice or following a dermatologist's routine or even quitting smoking. Few changed regimes will show instant results. More often than not, individuals have to persist with the change to see if it is having the desired effect.

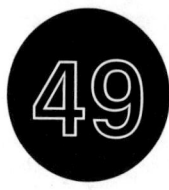

Stress

Stress is a factor that exacerbates many conditions. Whether it increases blood pressure or causes cardiovascular problems or even increases the intensity of acne flare-ups, stress is indeed something that is an avoidable part of our modern lives.

It is important to maintain stress levels at a minimum so that we may lead productive lives. Exercise, soothing music, yoga and other alternate therapies can reduce stress levels. It is advisable to minimize stress.

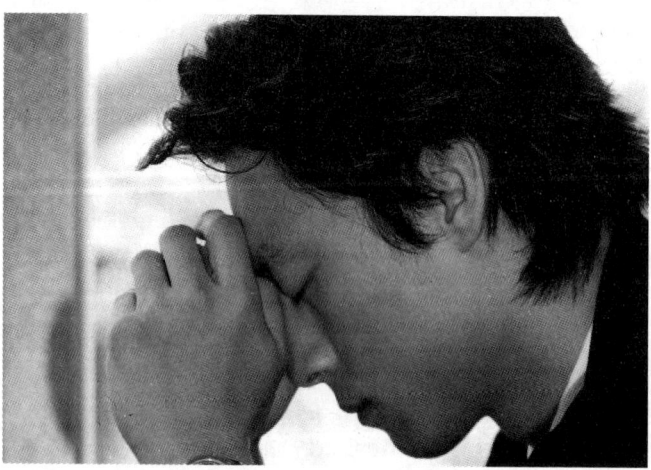

One study carried out in Singapore among adolescents showed a correlation between acne and stress. Despite the fact that there was no increase in the production of sebum during high stress periods (examination time) when compared to lower stress periods (vacations), the researchers found a positive correlation between stress and acne severity. Hence, it is essential to decrease stress levels to decrease the intensity of flare-ups.

Vitamin Deficiencies

It is essential for the human body to receive a recommended daily allowance of vitamins for its normal functioning. Vitamin deficiencies lead to many diseases and conditions, most of which are curable after the deficiency is noted and corrected.

The exact cause of acne is still debated but many factors that exacerbate the condition have been studied through decades. Some research studies have attributed that a lack of vitamins may aggravate acne. Vitamins

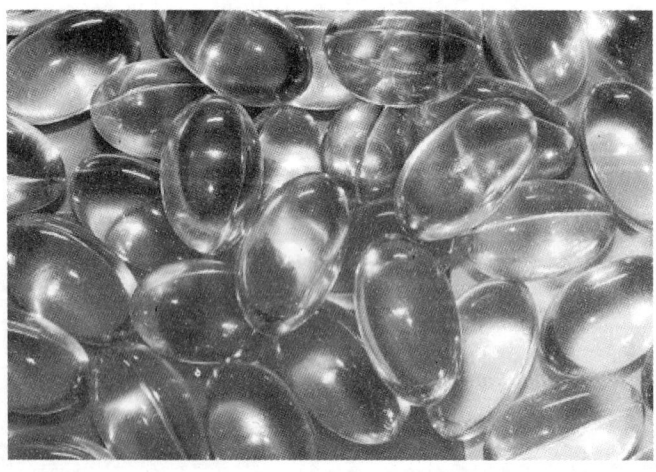

from all the major groups are essential for maintaining a healthy skin.

Vitamin A is very essential to maintain healthy skin. Derivatives of vitamin A are used by dermatologists to treat acne. Vitamins from the B complex group have been known since ages to help in maintaining clear skin. Studies on vitamin B_5 or panthothenic acid have shown that lack of this essential vitamin in certain diets leads to an aggravation of acne. One of the major functions both vitamin C and vitamin E is to mop up free radicals by acting as antioxidants. It is a proven fact that antioxidants help decrease the flare-up of acne. Vitamin D may also help in keeping the skin clear.

Hence, it is essential that vitamin deficiencies in the diet must be made up preferably by eating a balanced diet. Supplementation may be necessary but care must be taken as vitamin A, D, E and K at high levels are stored in the body mainly in the liver, and are toxic whereas excess of vitamins B and C are not stored by the body and are excreted.

Chapter 6
Treatment of Acne

Antibiotics

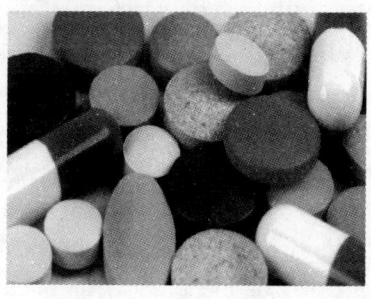

Antibiotics have been used by dermatologists to treat mild, moderate and severe cases of acne. Both topical for mild acne and oral antibiotics for moderate and severe acne have been used effectively on many individuals. However, some may not find antibiotics to be an effective treatment. Some affected persons have found that their initial bouts of acne have been treated effectively but recurring bouts seem to be totally unaffected by antibiotic treatment. This may be due to resistance developed as antibiotics treat the bacteria present on the skin and kill them or render them ineffective rather than addressing the root cause, of acne. Since there is no single root cause or there are multiple causes, each method of treatment has its own merits and demerits.

There are different types of antibiotics used to treat acne.

Topical Antibiotics

Topical antibiotics are used on the skin in the form of solutions, lotions or gels. Some are available on prescription. They are sometimes used in combination with benzoyl peroxide and/or topical retinoids.

Topical antibiotics may have side effects on susceptible individuals. These include dryness (combated by using a light water based moisturiser) or redness or itchiness due to a mild allergic reaction to the product (combated by using a topical steroid or hydrocortisone cream) or bacterial resistance due to infrequent use (combated by combining with benzoyl peroxide or topical retinoids). Hence most of the side effects can be dealt with by following the regular regime set by the dermatologist.

Oral Antibiotics

Oral antibiotics are generally taken as tablets and capsules. They are prescribed with a series of instructions and are taken before or after meals as per instructions prescribed.

Major oral antibiotics prescribed for acne are included from the following groups:

- Cotrimoxasole
- Erythromycin
- Tetracycline
- Trimethroprim

All these antibiotics may cause side effects in sensitive persons. They may cause allergies, photosensitivity, thrush, bacterial resistance and failure of the effectiveness of the contraceptive pill.

Recent studies have shown that rifampin was more effective when compared to other antibiotics. It was also suggested that a combination of rifampin with other antibiotics may improve the treatment. Researchers noted a synergistic effect between benzoyl peroxide and clindamycin or erythromycin.

Anti-inflammatories

Anti-inflammatories act on the surface of the skin. As their name suggests, they get rid of the inflammation including redness and swelling. Many anti-inflammatory agents are used topically as solutions or gels to treat mild and moderate acne. Some of the most common anti-inflammatory medicines including topical nicotinamide, naproxen, ibuprofen and calendula, are used to reduce the redness caused by acne.

Recent studies carried out using nicotinamide gel and clindamycin gel showed that both these gels in different concentrations were effective in reducing inflammation. It was also concluded that nicotinamide gel could be a preferable alternative to clindamycin gel as long time use of clindamycin may create resistance to treatment among certain acne prone individuals.

Benzoyl Peroxide

Benzoyl peroxide has been used from a long time to cure or reduce the symptoms of acne with a mild and moderate severity. It is also used along with antibiotics to decrease the acne of those who suffer from moderate to severe acne as research has proven its synergistic effect with certain antibiotics.

Researchers carried out double blind studies with benzoyl peroxide at concentrations of 2.5 per cent, 5 per cent and 10 per cent. They found that 2.5 per cent was as effective in reducing papules and pustules as other concentrations. After a topical application for two weeks, this concentration was also able to decrease the number of *propionibacterium acnes*. It also displayed less symptoms of burning and decreased the number of free fatty acids in the surface lipids.

When applied on the skin's surface, benzoyl peroxide breaks down to form oxygen and benzoic acid. Benzoic acid is a mild acid and oxygen is fatal for the anaerobic bacteria *Propionibacterium acnes*, the bacterium that thrives on the acne sufferer's skin. Benzoyl peroxide also has antiseptic and bleaching properties.

Benzoyl peroxide may also create mild irritation and dryness of the skin. It is always recommended that a person uses a light moisturiser along with this product. It should be used all over the skin surface and not just on spots. However, care should be taken to avoid the sensitive area around the eyes and also the hair which can get bleached on contact.

Some individuals who have extremely sensitive skin may find the dryness and irritation persisting. In such cases it is advisable to contact a dermatologist immediately and stop usage. In other cases it is advisable to start at low concentrations and if you find that its effects increase when you increase its concentration, it may be used in higher concentration till individual levels of tolerance are set.

Benzoyl peroxide is available in various forms including creams and gels, lotions and foams. It is available as soaps, medicated scrubs, face masks and face washes. This chemical is also an ingredient in various branded acne treatments.

Dermabrasion

Dermabrasion is a surgical procedure for removing the scarring caused by acne lesions. As the name suggests, the dermis (skin) is abraded (wearing away or rubbing a surface using friction). The upper layers of the skin (epidermis and dermis) are detached using a hand held electronic device. This procedure resurfaces the skin and effectively removes acne scars.

It has no effect on active acne and can in fact cause further infection. It is performed only on already present acne scars to decrease or remove them. In this procedure, conducted under local anaesthesia, a qualified plastic surgeon or dermatologist sloughs away the scarred and damaged tissues on the surface of the skin leaving behind the smoother and newer skin below to slowly grow and heal naturally and stay clear.

Dermabrasion has few side effects and its results are not seen immediately. It has proven to have had mixed results with some people strongly advocating its utility and others believing that it has not had much effect on their acne.

It is essential to note that this procedure should be done under the supervision of or by well qualified personnel for optimum results. Otherwise there may be complications. After care instructions should be followed thoroughly and the dermatologist or surgeon should be consulted immediately if there are any adverse reactions.

Dermabrasion is quite expensive and may require several sittings as recommended by the dermatologist. It is only recommended for removing scarred tissue and not to prevent the outbreak of new acne lesions. It is generally used for moderate to severe cases of acne.

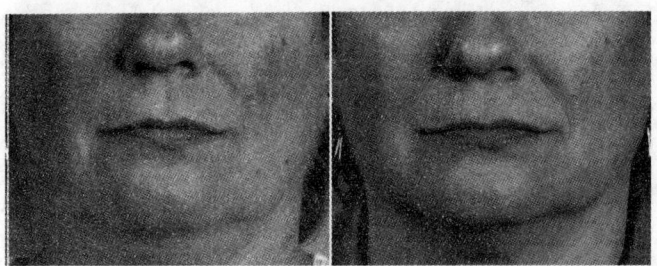

For milder cases, microdermabrasion, a gentler and less invasive procedure is used. In this procedure, the thin outer layer of the skin is removed without the need of anaesthetics. It is a milder procedure which may be performed at home with self-help kits which may or may not give you good results. It can also be performed by dermatologists, at beauty salons and spas.

Pilot studies on microdermabrasion show that this procedure has a positive effect in improving acne scars.

Hormonal Treatment

Since it has been proven that androgens or male hormones play a role in exacerbating acne flare-ups in some individuals, it goes without saying that treating these individuals by balancing the production of these hormones will decrease their outbreaks of acne.

Hormonal treatment is useful for those women who suffer from moderate to severe attacks of acne. Initially tests are conducted to confirm that there are elevated levels of androgens produced in the body. When elevated results are found, treatment begins to lower the androgen activity thus eliminating the cause of acne. Properly planned hormonal treatment under the supervision of trained and experienced gynaecologists and endocrinologists have shown good results even when people have had fairly severe cystic acne. Hormonal treatment is fairly individualistic and needs medical supervision. It is essential that you regulate your hormones after consulting a specialist.

Hormones are regulated using two types of medications:

1. Oral Contraceptive Pills

This is one of the most effective ways of treating acne as these pills decrease the production of testosterone that leads to a decrease in androgen production which finally results in a decrease in acne. Despite its easy availability, some contraceptives have side effects. They include spotting, nausea, dizziness, loss of or increase in appetite, headaches and mood changes. Hence, it is advisable to consult a specialist rather than self-medicating.

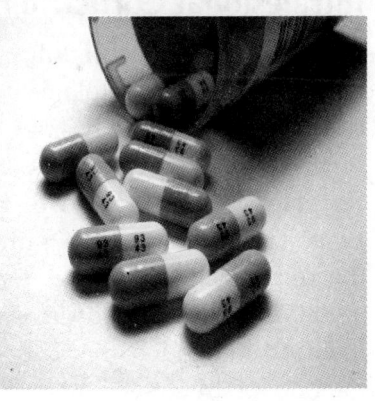

Studies on the use of different combinations of contraceptive pills have been carried out by several researchers and they report that oral contraceptives have been found to be effective in treating adult acne in women.

2. Spironolactone

Spironolactone is a synthetic steroid that binds with androgen receptors and reduces its synthesis thus decreasing androgen levels in the body. It also has various side effects including nausea, diarrhoea, dizziness, drowsiness, headaches and irregular menstrual cycles. As with other medications, it is advisable to use this method of treatment under medical supervision.

Intralesional Corticosteroid Injections

For severe cases of adult acne when large cysts are present, dermatologists recommend injecting corticosteroids directly into the cyst. This results in flattening of acne cysts. There is some ongoing research on this method of treating severe cases of acne. This is done on a purely individual basis on the recommendation of a dermatologist when other methods to cure or decrease the acne have failed. It is recommended that this should not be the sole method of treatment as long term consequences of the corticosteroid injections have not been sufficiently studied. There are a few side effects and this treatment does not address the other underlying causes of acne and may even cause steroid induced acne

Studies on the use of **triamcinolone acetonide** by researchers to treat cystic lesions proved that they were effective in the treatment of cystic acne and further trials were recommended. Later pilot studies have shown a combination therapy of triamcinolone acetonide with lincomycin were more effective than using only triamcinolone acetonide. Further studies are needed to find the lowest concentrations needed to promote their synergistic effect.

As with other acne treatments, an individual's response to various treatments is varied. Always consult a good dermatologist and don't self-medicate unless you have very mild acne.

Laser

Laser treatment has been used since quite a while to get rid of acne scars. However, there is insufficient data on the efficacy of its use. No long term studies have been carried out on the effects of laser on acne scarring and generally with current studies, the sample sizes have been small in number.

Mixed data has been collected by different researchers on the effectiveness of laser beams on acne scarred skin tissue. Many users also post conflicting opinions as some believe that it has helped with their scarring while others feel that it is a waste of time and money. Some patients have reported the recurrence of acne while others have found that they have achieved better results after laser treatment in combination with topical prescription skin ointments.

Treatment of acne scars by laser beams is an expensive process. It requires several sittings and is preferably done by a qualified dermatologist rather than at beauty spas and beauty salons. Care should be taken that experienced and qualified personnel use the equipment. There are side effects including the formation of blisters, hyper pigmentation and excessive dryness of the skin. As with other treatments, an individual having acne prone skin may react differently depending upon the individual's, severity of acne and his/her sensitivity.

Phototherapy

Light has been used from time immemorial to heal. It is an essential factor for good health as sunlight provides the essential 'sunshine vitamin' or vitamin D. Sunlight in limited amounts is good for skin and dry heat from the skin has a protective effect on the skin. Recent research on light has shown the positive effect of single bands of light like blue light or red light or a combination of both to be beneficial in curing or at least decreasing acne.

Phototherapy is considered to be an effective method to treat acne vulgaris. It is a non-invasive procedure and generally there is no recovery time as with other surgical or chemical procedures. Generally regarded as safe, phototherapy is not recommended for those who are light sensitive or those who suffer from epilepsy.

Several sessions of phototherapy are required and may prove to be expensive. In recent times, phototherapy is also available in the form of home portable units. However, care should be taken and instructions should be followed carefully.

Studies carried out using a narrow band blue light source on people with mild and moderate acne showed that the acne lesions reduced considerably over a period of time and caused no adverse side effects. Only two people experienced dryness but they continued with the treatment.

Studies carried out on mild to moderate sufferers of acne with blue light, blue and red light combined and white light showed that the final improvement in acne comedones was more significant when a combination of blue and red light therapy was used. The researchers concluded that the combination of antibacterial and anti-inflammatory action of blue and red light therapy treated mild to moderate acne activity and left no significant unfavourable effects.

Phototherapy has proved to be effective in decreasing acne vulgaris in short term studies without any discernible side effects. However it must be noted that many long term studies have not been carried out using phototherapy.

Retinoids

Topical

Topical retinoids are synthetic derivatives of vitamin A. They are generally used to treat mild cases of acne and are sometimes combined with other treatments to treat moderate and severe cases of acne. Topical retinoids are available in the form of gels, creams and liquids. They include adapalene, tretinoin and tazarotene.

Topical retinoids should be used judiciously and instructions should be followed carefully as many people who use them suffer from side effects including dryness or redness of skin which disappears after a while. It is advisable not to apply retinoids at the time when one applies **benzoyl peroxide**. It is also essential to stay away from sunlight and retinoids are generally applied in the evenings. When there are severe side effects, it is a must to immediately discontinue its use and to consult a dermatologist. **Retinoids** are counter indicated during pregnancy.

Studies by various researchers have shown that topical retinoids can significantly treat inflammatory acne. However it has been noticed that in clinical practice these retinoids are also used to treat non-inflammatory acne.

Some retinoids are available over the counter. Despite the fact that retinoids may be available easily, it is always advisable to get it as prescribed medicine as wrong usage or less potent medications maybe the ones more easily available but they also may be the ones that finally prove to be less effective or have unknown adverse side effects as well.

Oral

Oral retinoids are used to treat severe cases of acne including nodular and cystic acne. Isotretinoin is the derivative of vitamin A used to treat the condition. The exact mechanism on how it inhibits cystic acne is unknown. However it is said to decrease sebum production and has an antimicrobial action on *Propionibacterium acnes*.

As with other acne treatments, it has its side effects which may be stronger than other medications. Hence it is considered more as a final treatment and used more often to cure severe acne although it is sometimes used as treatment for moderate cases. It is available in some countries and through the internet without prescription. It is dangerous to use it without a prescription as it has well documented side effects. It should be used under the medical supervision of a dermatologist as a number of side effects are reported as a result of its use.

However, many cases of severe acne have been cleared up after the use of isotretinoin. Just as there are various success stories attributed to the use of this retinoids there are also various complications and adverse side effects noted when it is used. It has been implicated in causing birth defects, depression, etc. Thus, the advice of a dermatologist is essential as the dosage, the precautions and the completion of the course of treatment with isotretinoin is extremely important.

Several studies have shown that the chemical is an effective treatment for severe cases of acne under medical supervision. A ten year study on isotretinoin in Singapore concluded that this derivate is effective for severe acne and there was a remission in a major number of cases. It also recommended lower dosages for decreasing its adverse effects.

Salicylic Acid

Salicylic acid is natural phytohormone found in several plant sources. Acetyl salicylic acid is also known as aspirin. Salicylic acid has been used as an anti-inflammatory agent since ancient times to cure aches and pains, and fevers. Its anti-inflammatory action has made it useful as a treatment for acne. It reduces swelling and redness. It can unplug the skin pores causing the pimples to shrink in size. Some mild irritation or dryness may be seen as a side effect. It is better to inform and consult your doctor or dermatologist if you have any severe side effects.

It can be used as a topical preparation. It is often used in OTC topical preparations and is available as cream, gel, lotion and liquid. It is also available as cloth pads and wipes.

Research studies on the use of salicylic acid pads to treat mild and moderate acne showed that these pads decreased the number of primary lesions thus decreasing the number and severity of all the lesions present. A few patients suffered from mild skin irritation. However, as with any treatment, care must be taken to see that the acne sufferer does not react adversely to salicylic acid or its derivatives. If adverse effects are noted, discontinue immediately as some people are sensitive to its use.

Studies on salicylic acid peels to treat acne vulgaris in Asian women were conducted. The studies confirmed that the peels were effective in reducing inflammatory and non-inflammatory acne lesions and the side effects were tolerated by most of the women.

Sulphur

Sulphur has been used to treat skin disorders from time immemorial and is one of the oldest known naturally occurring mineral to treat acne. It is present in our bodies in miniscule quantities. Sulphur baths, also called **balneotherapy** have been used to treat various skin conditions.

Topical sulphur, in the form of cream, lotion and gel, has been used to treat mild and moderate forms of acne. It does not seem to have much effect on severe acne. It takes a few weeks to see results but many acne sufferers have seen positive effects after the judicious use of sulphur based products.

Sulphur is considered to be an exfoliating agent and peels away dead cells. It is also said to have a mild antiseptic action. It may reduce oiliness. It may also produce side effects including redness of skin, itchiness and irritation. Sulphur has a strong odour. Some people may be allergic to sulphur and sulphur compounds.

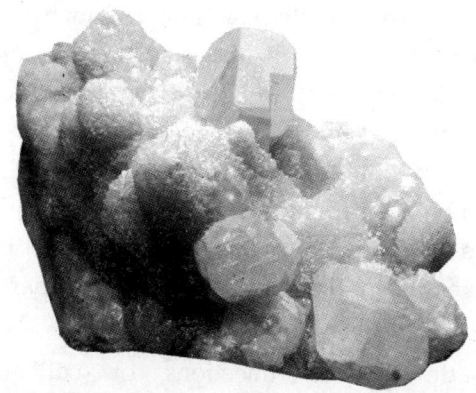

Sulphur is used both as a single ingredient and in combination with other chemicals like **benzoyl peroxide**, resorcinol and salicylic acid. It is available as both OTC and prescription drug.

Researchers found that a combination of benzoyl peroxide with sulphur gave good to excellent results on people undergoing this treatment with few people suffering minimal side effects of tightness and drying of skin.

Surgery

When severe acne in the form of deep cysts, severe inflammation, extensively damaged skin and lots of scarring is present, surgery may be performed by a very well qualified dermatologist as a last resort when all conventional treatments have failed. Punch excisions and skin graftings are only undertaken in serious cases. They require expertise and are generally undertaken under constant medical supervision for large and deep scars by qualified plastic surgeons. Punch grafts may also be used to get rid of scars. It is advisable to discuss all the pros and cons of any surgical method undertaken as anaesthesia is an important part of the procedure.

Sometimes filler injections of collagen by dermatologists are used to treat depressed acne scars. This treatment has evoked a mixed response and most users find it a temporary measure to get rid of scars while other adults feel that it has decreased their scars and improved their skin. As with other treatment methods, filling in collagen to treat acne scars has its pluses and minuses.

Surgical lancing under the guidance of qualified surgeons, to allow the pus to escape from abscesses, may also be performed if necessary.

Other Treatments

Several conventional, natural, alternate and holistic treatments have also been used to treat the various forms of acne. Although these may be considered to be generally less harmful, care should be taken as the human body can be as allergic to natural compounds as it is to artificial ones. There is no guarantee that a natural, holistic treatment will have more or less effect than an allopathic western treatment.

Each treatment has its own advantages and disadvantages. Very often, a combination of treatments has shown to work when treating acne through western or allopathic treatment. This may hold true with natural treatments as well. There are so many possibilities of treatment working or not working individually that it is difficult to compare treatments.

The only fact that has been established as far as treatments is considered is that western or allopathic treatment takes quite a while, at least four weeks and may even take twelve weeks to show that they work.

Some of the alternative treatments include:

Acupressure or Acupuncture

Acupressure may also be called **Shiatsu massage**. Fingertips and thumb are used to massage or manipulate certain specific pressure points on the face or body. The ancient Chinese believed that two life forces—Yang (active force) and Yin (passive force) govern the general health of the body. When these forces are not synchronized, different parts of the body get imbalanced. By applying pressure on specific points these imbalances are removed and the Chi or life force now flows through the meridian (nerve like channels), maintaining a balance in the body.

When fine needles are used to channelize the Chi through these meridians, the technique is called **acupuncture**.

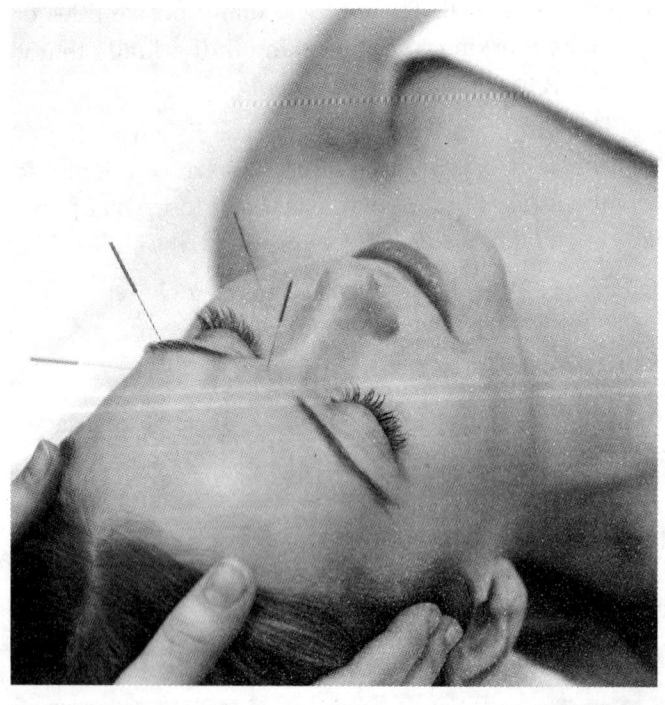

Aloe Vera

Aloe vera is an ancient medicinal plant. It has been used to treat various skin conditions. It has an anti-inflammatory action. It is used in various forms like juice, gel and capsule. It is also used in formulating creams and soaps.

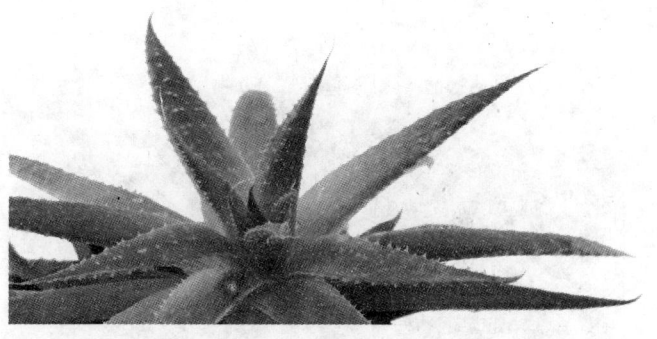

Aloe vera is said to improve skin and heal acne marks and scars. One can apply the fresh sap or gel from the leaves topically on acne scars. Applied topically, aloe vera cream has had modest to good benefits among a wide variety of users. However, it does not cure or prevent acne flare-ups. It may be applied topically after cleaning the face. It has a good effect on most skins but some people may find that it has no benefit or that it does not suit their skin.

Aromatherapy

Aromatherapy may be used to treat acne. There has been some research on the benefits of tea tree oil in treating acne. It is said to possess anti-bacterial, anti-fungal and anti-viral properties. It has a strong and distinct smell which reminds one of disinfectants.

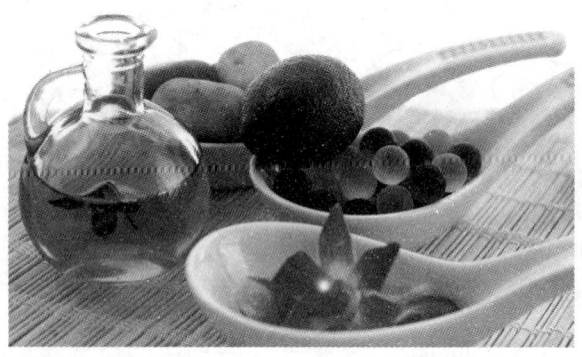

Tea tree oil is the most common essential oil used to treat acne. It is obtained by steam distillation of the leaves of a native Australian tree *Melaleuca alternifolia*. One study said that tea tree oil was as effective as benzoyl peroxide in treating acne though the duration of treatment could be longer. There were fewer side effects including itchiness, dryness, etc. when compared to benzoyl peroxide. However tea tree oil does not cure acne. Some skins may be sensitive to its application so it is always advisable to try it out in very small quantities.

Other aromatic oils that may be used to treat acne include jasmine essential oil, lavender essential oil, myrrh essential oil, sandalwood essential oil and ylang ylang essential oil. After sufficient dilution, blends of aromatic oil may be directly applied to the surface of the skin or inhaled through steam in very small quantities.

Ayurvedic Treatment for Acne

As per ayurveda, acne is called **'yauvan pidika'** as it often affects youth or adolescents. It is considered as an internal disturbance of the body. Improper diet and faulty eating habits are believed to be the cause of yauvan pidika.

To treat acne, the ayurvedic form of treatment uses a specific diet, hygiene (a daily bath), exposure to sunlight and fresh air, certain herbs and exercise.

Azelaic Acid

Azelaic acid is a natural dicarboxylic acid present in grains like wheat, barley and rye. It has an anti-bacterial action. It may be used to treat mild and moderate acne–comedonal and inflammatory forms of acne. It is able to reduce inflammation and hence it may be used to treat acne rosacea.

Studies have proved its efficacy at treating the condition at 20 per cent cream formulation and at 15 per cent gel form. However it must be noted that some people find this acid to be a skin irritant. In combination with zinc sulphate, azelaic acid can be a good method of treating androgen related (hormonal) activity of the skin.

Black Currant Seed Oil

Black currant seed oil is a rich source of essential fatty acids, vitamin C and many minerals. It is widely available in the form of tablets, creams and gels.

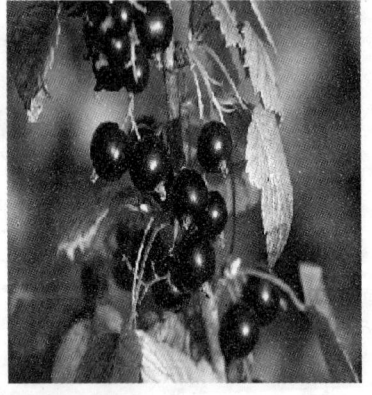

It has an anti-inflammatory action. It has proven to be effective in treating skin conditions including acne. It must be noted that excessive use of black currant seed oil can cause arthritis. So do consult your dermatologist before thinking of self-medication.

Chinese Herbal Medicine

Chinese herbal medicine is an entire field of treatment by itself and like other alternative methods, some acne sufferers believe that it can and has cured acne. Several capsules which are a mixture of herbs are available to cure acne.

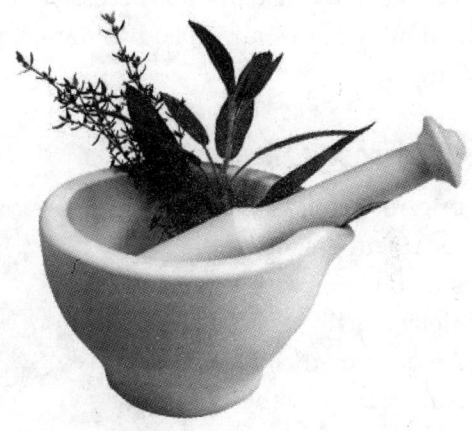

Generally complementary herbs together with diet control are used by Chinese herbalists.

Cod Liver Oil

Cod liver oil or oils from fatty fish are generally considered healthy. They are good sources of essential fatty acids including omega-3 fatty acids. It is believed that the eicosapentaenoic acid or EPA present in fish oils inhibits androgen activity. Since hormonal activity, especially that of androgen has been isolated as a major cause of acne in some individuals, it may be the reason why fish oils help in decreasing acne.

It must be noted that indiscriminate use of fish oil supplements is inadvisable as excess of oil even in the form of essential fatty acids is not necessary for the normal functioning of the human body and may prove to be detrimental.

Evening Primrose Oil

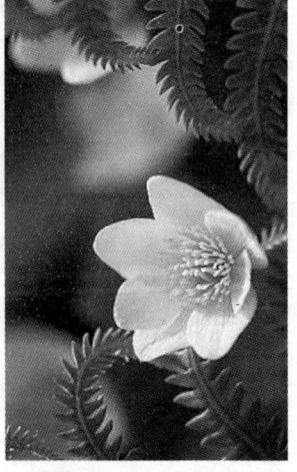

Evening primrose oil is a good source of many essential fatty acids mainly GLA or gamma linoleic acid. It is considered to be a medicinal plant and is used to treat and heal various conditions. It is stated to have some effect on reducing acne flare-ups as it is anti-inflammatory in action.

It may reduce sebum production. Thus it reduces clogging of pores. It has a calm and soothing effect on dry, itchy, red skin. It may help those who suffer from acne rosacea. Topical application of the oil has given promising results to some sufferers of acne in reducing flare-ups. It cannot treat acne.

Flaxseed Oil

Flaxseed oil is a rich source of essential fatty acids. Sufferers of acne have shown mixed reactions to using this natural food as a supplement to cure acne. Some have benefitted while others have found their acne worsening.

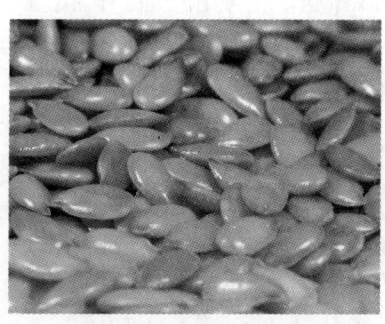

Flaxseeds may be consumed either as seeds (golden or brown) or as oil in capsules.

Homoeopathy

In homoeopathy there are certain treatments for acne. Generally the homoeopath individually studies each acne sufferer and recommends treatment.

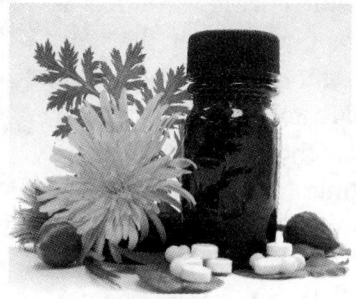

Treatment includes the use of belladonna, calendula officinalis, silicea. terra, hepar sulphuris and kalium bromatum depending upon the type of pustules formed.

Some acne sufferers have reported that homoeopathy helped them to reduce their acne. As with other holistic and natural treatments, the choice of using homoeopathy is left to the individual.

Lemon Juice and Cucumber

A combination of fresh lemon juice and cucumber has been used to lighten acne scars. Generally lemon juice is not applied directly on the skin as it is astringent in nature and causes a stinging reaction. When combined with cucumber it has a cooling effect on the skin. Lemon combined with cucumber juice is applied on the scars for a short time (depending on the individual from ten minutes up to half an hour) and then the face is gently washed with water.

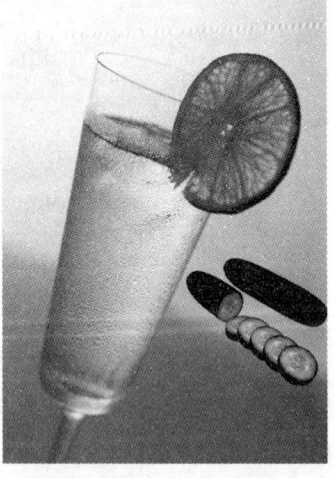

Olive Leaf Extract

The olive tree is considered to be an ancient and blessed tree by many civilizations. Every part of this tree has found use and the health benefits from the olive tree are well documented. Hence, it is not surprising to know that extracts from the olive leaf help to reduce acne in some individuals. The leaves are supposed to have antiseptic and astringent properties.

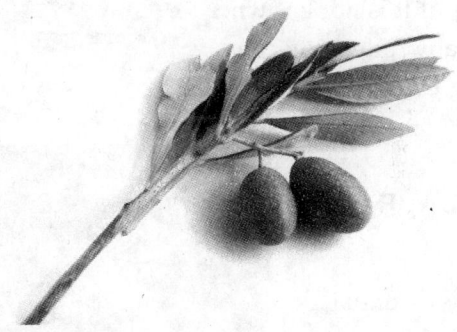

However it must be remembered that some people may be allergic to the extract and if any side effects like headache, nausea, etc. manifests after use, it is advisable to discontinue it.

Reflexology

When pressure is applied to certain points generally on the feet, the process is termed as reflexology.

Some people say that they have found relief from acne outbursts when reflexology has been used to balance their liver or endocrine systems. As with other holistic treatments, this may or may not suit all individuals. It may work as a placebo or as a temporary treatment but it is not known if it has any effect on the underlying cause of the acne flare-up.

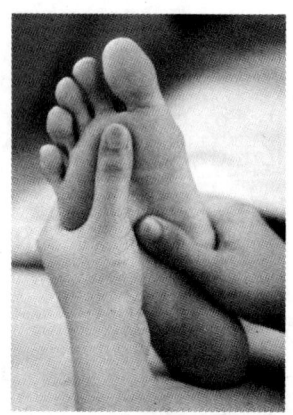

Vitamins A, B_5 and E

Vitamin A is essential for the normal functioning of the skin. Several derivatives of vitamin A are used in topical and oral applications to treat acne. Vitamin A supplements may be good provided one does not overdose

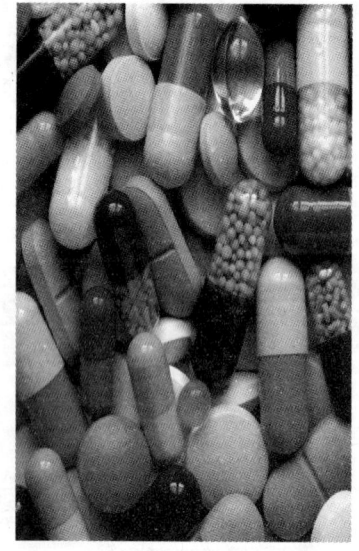

as the vitamin can get stored in the body and cause toxicity.

Vitamin B_5 or pantothenic acid helps to balance hormones which are considered to be a major cause of acne in many individuals. It also decreases stress and it is a known fact that while stress does not cause acne it can increase the severity of acne flare-ups. There is generally no toxicity as excess of all vitamins from the B complex group are normally excreted from the body. However, it is always advisable not to take an overdose of any vitamin.

Vitamin E

Vitamin E has antioxidant properties and antioxidants help to treat acne. Excessive intake of vitamin E is inadvisable.

Yoga

Yoga is a form of relaxation with general benefits as well as specific benefits. Certain yogic postures help the body to go into deep relaxation eliminating a lot of stress from the body.

Yoga may benefit people who have acne under the guidance of yoga teachers as certain yogic postures are designed specifically for the face. It may also balance hormonal imbalances. Yoga may also improve general

142 | 50 Things That Cause Acne

health thus benefitting the skin and decreasing acne flare-ups.

Yoga should be practiced under the guidance of a qualified teacher.

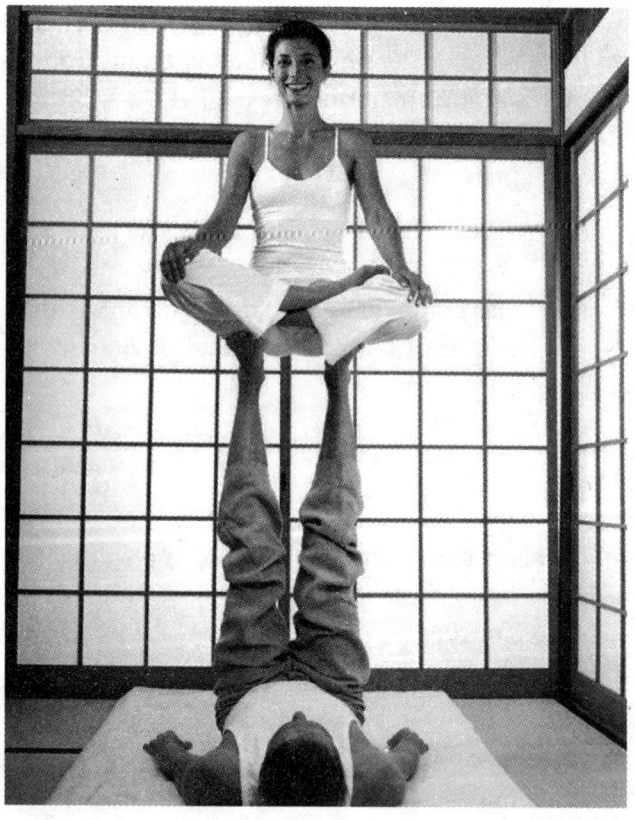

Zinc

Zinc is an essential mineral which may help to treat acne in many individuals. It is present in many foods. As a supplement, it has been found effective in treating acne in several individuals. However, zinc cannot cure acne. There is no single cure for acne.

Studies on the efficacy of zinc gluconate regimens for three months proved that they were effective in reducing inflammatory acne.

Chapter 7

Management of Acne

Management for Mild Acne

It is generally simple and easy to treat mild cases of acne. It is necessary to wash the face and other affected areas twice daily with a mild soap.

Topical ointments including topical retinoids or topical benzoyl peroxide may be used. It takes a few weeks for the treatment to have an effect. It is important to avoid exposure to the sun when certain formulations, especially retinoids are used. Generally four to eight weeks is the normal period of treatment for mild acne. There may be some dryness and initial irritation. If it persists or is severe, please contact a dermatologist.

Management for Moderate Acne

Treatment for moderate acne includes topical retinoids, benzoyl peroxide and topical antibiotics that may be used to curb inflammation. The treatment may vary between six weeks to eight weeks. If there are severe rashes or inflammation, it is essential to contact a dermatologist. Some amount of maintenance treatment may also be necessary.

Management for Severe Acne

Together with topical medicines, oral antibiotics and hormones may be prescribed. It is essential that the acne sufferer is under the care of a dermatologist. Treatment with antibiotics may continue for up to twelve weeks or more and it needs the constant supervision of a dermatologist. Medication may continue for a long period to maintain the reduction of acne.

Management for Very Severe Acne

Very severe acne can be treated only by a dermatologist as no topical or over the counter medicine generally has any effect. Isotretinoin is the main line of treatment and is expensive. It has to be used correctly to have maximum effect. Sometimes other treatments including antibiotics and hormonal treatments may be added by the qualified dermatologist. The treatment period may vary and needs to be continued as per the specialists' instruction up to a period of six months.

Tips

Healthy Diet

A long time ago a lawyer called Brillat Savarin said "Tell me what you eat and I will tell you who you are." He was also the author of the famous book *Physiologie du gout* or the *Physiology of Taste* first published in 1825. This adage still holds true after centuries.

According to our elders, today we consume more junk food. I believe that there is no such thing as junk food but there is healthy food which can be consumed as much we can and unhealthy food which gives us satiety value and sometimes elevates our moods but such foods must be eaten in small quantities.

Our body is a sensitive yet hard working machine which works well when we give it the correct fuel. It is important to eat healthy foods to keep the body fit. Some studies have shown that acne prone people also benefit when they eat healthy diets. Another aspect to be considered as far as food is concerned is that some individuals are sensitive to certain foods which may cause allergic reactions where inflammation is a result and this might just exacerbate acne.

Studies conducted by researchers have shown that a diet that has a low glycemic load had improved acne and insulin sensitivity in male acne patients. The researchers felt that further studies were necessary.

Other studies also found that there was a great difference in the incidence of acne between westernized societies and non-westernized societies. They postulated that it was not only hereditary and genetic factors but also environmental factors including traditional healthy eating patterns that led to the zero incidence of acne in such rural and fairly isolated societies that were studied.

So a healthy diet filled with fruits and vegetables, whole grains and good quality proteins may help you control your acne.

Water

Water is an essential nutrient for the normal functioning of the human body. Among several others, one of the main functions of water is to flush out toxins from the body. Drinking sufficient water, up to 2 litres in temperate climates and up to 3 litres in the tropics, especially during summer is advisable. Water is a cleanser, purifier and stabilizer as it maintains the balance in the body.

However do not overdo on water consumption as high levels of water can be toxic and the fact that water intoxication causes imbalances in the body is a researched fact. Consuming water or liquids throughout the day is advisable rather than consuming

Management of Acne | 149

large volumes together to maintain both the water and the sodium-potassium balance in the body.

Exercise

Without regular exercise, the human body resembles an old inefficient machine which plods along perhaps due to a good and intelligent design rather than regular maintenance. Just as we take care of so many inanimate but important gizmos in our life like mobile phones, computers and other hi-fi equipment by regularly charging them and cleaning them, it is essential that we maintain our bodies with regular exercise.

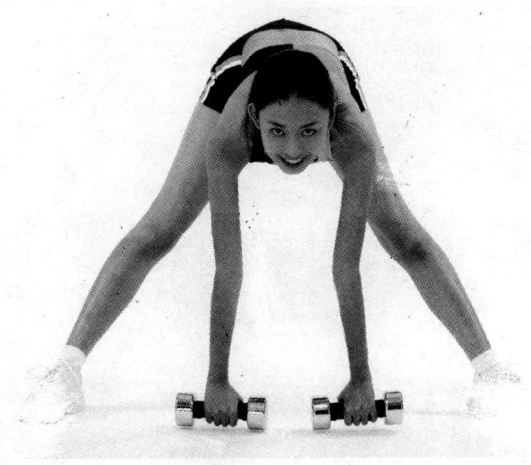

Exercise is to the body what prayer or meditation is to the soul. It keeps the body in ship-shape condition and makes life good. A regular bout of exercise is uplifting for both the body and the mind. It also helps to keep the skin clear. Hence, it can definitely help acne prone individuals to maintain good health. As wise men have said 'health is wealth.' By being healthy and having a clear skin one can even decrease the amount of money spent for acne treatments some of which are expensive!

Regular Cleansing Routine

A regular cleansing routine including washing one's face twice a day with a mild soap is absolutely essential to prevent further acne breakouts. Washing the skin can remove dead skin cells and excess of oil that may be present

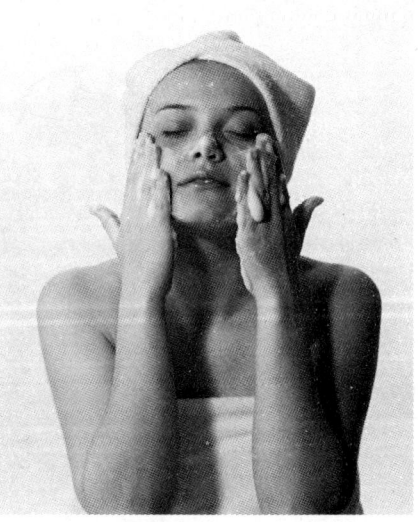

on the surface of the skin. However, cleaning the face too often is inadvisable as it may increase inflammation and irritate the already sensitive skin. Rare cleaning of the face is also detrimental as this may also increase the clogging of pores and cause accumulation of dead cells and excess oil. Hence, it has been laid down as a rule that cleaning the face twice daily is a good cleansing routine. Acne products have to be applied on clean skin. If you feel a stinging sensation or burning sensation after you apply the product, wait for about ten minutes after washing your face and then apply the product.

Regular Shampooing

Excess of oil on the skin may also lead to oily hair. It is advisable to wash hair daily with a mild shampoo to decrease the oiliness and avoid the possibility of the hairline or scalp getting affected with acne.

Dandruff has been implicated as a factor that aggravates acne as they have a similar aetiology. It is advisable to treat the scalp if you have excess dandruff as this will help decrease your acne outbreaks.

Squeezing or Picking Blemishes

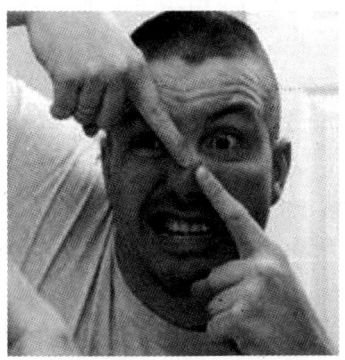

It is totally inadvisable to pop, pick or squeeze blemishes, especially acne lesions which are inflammatory. The infected material in these lesions will be pushed further inside the skin increasing inflammation and may even increase the scarring of the skin.

Use Oil Free Products

It is a known fact that excess of sebum (oil) production is one of the major causes of acne. Therefore it goes without saying that the oil production in the body or the surface of the skin should remain minimal. Thus, it is advisable to use oil-free products. There are many oil-free, non-comedogenic products available in the market. They are generally expensive but may be worth the price of reducing rather than increasing the acne on your face, if they suit you.

Certain Healthy Foods

Blueberries

Blueberries are small but power packed houses of nutrition. They contain enough vital vitamins and minerals to be among the healthier berries available to humankind. They are good sources of antioxidants which are essential for the normal functioning of the body as they mop up free radicals produced as a result of many of the metabolic activities of the body. Free radicals are capable of damaging the normal functioning of the body. A diet rich in antioxidants is essential for normal health. This diet has also proven to be good to combat acne.

Many foods contain antioxidants. However, blueberries have a fairly large amount of them in combination with other essential vitamins and minerals. It is easily possible to add fresh blueberries to one's diet and many acne sufferers have noticed a favourable change in their skin with bouts of acne decreasing and almost disappearing.

Blueberries have also been effective in combination with other fruits as fruit juices. It is also effectively used as a face pack. However, avoid too much consumption of any single food in your diet.

Brewer's Yeast

The connection between brewer's yeast and acne is generally considered as a beneficial one. However, some individuals may be allergic to brewer's yeast. Brewer's yeast may also react with other medications. Before supplementing the diet with brewer's yeast, it is important to discuss its effects with your physician, dermatologist or pharmacist.

Supplements of brewer's yeast have cleared up the skin of many acne prone individuals. Studies conducted on volunteers suffering from different types of acne showed that around 80 per cent of them who were administered a nutritional supplement of brewer's yeast showed fairly remarkable changes in their skin with it becoming clearer and with lesser blemishes.

Brewer's yeast is a combination of different strains of yeasts. It is a cocktail of many essential vitamins and minerals including those from the B complex group and zinc. It is available as powder, as flakes and also as both tablets and capsules and is generally taken after meals. It has a fairly unpalatable taste and smell.

However, it is important to note that excessive use of brewer's yeast leads to many side effects and complications including breathlessness, itchy skin, development of rashes, headaches, a bloated feeling, nausea, diarrhoea and excessive gas production.

As with most natural products, it is very important to note that excessive dosages of the product may even exacerbate the acne due to the production of rashes. It is always advisable to start with minimum quantities and to slowly increase the dosage to one's tolerance levels. It is also a major ingredient in many face creams.

Cranberries

Cranberries are a good source of antioxidants, vitamins and minerals. They have shown to be beneficial in decreasing the symptoms of acne outbursts.

Cranberries are more often than not consumed as a fruit juice. When you use cranberry juice, be sure to read the label so that you consume the actual juice without any added sugar. Added sugar has no value except to provide more calories. In fact, sugar has been implicated in causing or aggravating acne in many individuals.

If possible, it is better to eat fresh and raw berries as one gets to consume fibre and other beneficial factors in the fruit which get destroyed during its processing.

Pumpkin

It is indeed a rare case that an individual may be prone to acne after consuming pumpkin, as generally pumpkin pulp and pumpkin seeds are associated more with the clearing and cleansing of the skin due to the optimum amounts of both zinc and essential fatty acids present in them.

Glossary

Abscess
A group of pus cells in any part of the body, containing pus formed by bacterial action and often followed by inflammation around these cells.

Acupressure
Applying pressure using one's fingers at specific points in the body.

Acupuncture
Piercing specific areas of the body with fine needles to relieve pain or other symptoms.

Alternative Therapies
Healing practices that are different from conventional western therapies.

Alzheimer's Disease

The most common form of dementia where patients undergo confusion, mood swings, memory loss, etc.

Anabolic Steroids

Drugs that copy the effects of male androgens including testosterone and dihydrotestosterone.

Androgens

A group of hormones, found predominantly in males, involved in the growth and development of their reproductive system.

Antibiotics

Substances or compounds that kill bacteria or inhibit their growth.

Anticonvulsants

Drugs that prevent convulsions and seizures often used to treat epilepsy.

Anti-inflammatories

Foods, drugs or substances used to reduce inflammation.

Aromatherapy

A form of alternative medicine that uses essential oils and aromatic substances to promote physical and psychological well being.

Ayurveda

A traditional Indian medical system used to treat different kinds of diseases and conditions.

Azelaic acid

An anti-bacterial acid found naturally in wheat, barley and rye, used to treat inflammations.

Barbiturates

These drugs act on the central nervous system to decrease anxiety or induce sleep.

Blackhead

It consists of a blackened plug of sebum, skin debris and bacteria that clogs a pore in the skin.

Capsaicin

A colourless and pungent crystalline compound obtained from capsicum or chillies.

Chinese Herbal Medicine

An alternative therapy where traditional Chinese herbs are used to cure different types of ailments and conditions.

Chronic

A persistent or long lasting condition or disease.

Comedones

Closed or open hair follicles consisting of sebum, skin debris and bacteria that clog skin pores.

Convulsions

A medical condition where the body muscles shake uncontrollably and rapidly due to contraction and relaxation.

Curcumin

The principal natural compound present in turmeric that is well known for its healing properties.

Cyst

An abnormal blister or sac that contains a solid, semisolid or liquid substance inside it.

DHEA

An endogenous steroid said to improve growth and muscle and sold as a dietary supplement in some countries.

Dermabrasion

A surgical procedure where upper layers of the skin are removed; the procedure is used to remove acne scars.

Dermatologist

A medical expert who treats common and uncommon skin disorders.

Dermis

Dermis is the layer of skin between the epidermis and the subcutaneous tissue.

Endocrinologist

A medical specialist who treats problems related to the endocrine system (the complex system of hormones).

Epidermis

It is the outer layer of skin.

Essential Fatty Acids

These fatty acids are essential for the normal functioning of the human body. They cannot be manufactured by the body and need to be provided in the daily diet.

Exacerbate

To make conditions more intense and aggravating.

Glycemic index (GI)

The glycemic index of foods is a measurement of how quickly different carbohydrates are broken down to glucose and released into the blood.

Hispanics

People from Spain or Spanish speaking countries in Latin America.

Homoeopathy

A system of medicine developed by Dr Hahnemann that treats conditions and diseases on the principle of 'like cures like.'

Inflammation

A response of the body to irritation or injury with redness, swelling, tenderness, etc.

Isoflavones

They are phytoestrogens, natural hormone-like plant derivatives that are present in soya bean.

Laser

A source of high intensity light radiation (infra red, ultraviolet, etc.) produced by stimulated emission.

Nodules

A small hard mass of tissues found on the skin of acne patients.

Obesity

Excess of body fat accumulated; it often has an adverse effect on the health and well being of the individual.

Oral

Taken or ingested through the mouth.

Papules

Small and rounded elevations, sometimes inflammatory, found on the skin.

Pilosebaceous Unit

The hair, hair follicle and sebaceous glands are called a pilosebaceous unit.

Phototherapy

Treating conditions of the skin using ultra violet or infra red rays.

Pimple

When the skin's pores get blocked, pimples are formed.

Pustules

A cavity on the skin filled with pus cells.

Reflexology

A massage to relieve pain using finger pressure on the feet.

Retinoid

A natural derivative of vitamin A found in the body in small quantities.

Salicylic Acid

A white acid mostly commonly used to make aspirin.

Satiety

The state of being satisfied or a feeling of fullness after eating food.

Sebum

An oily substance secreted by the sebaceous glands.

Seborrhea

A condition where one has red or flaky skin.

Seizures

A sudden attack, spasm or convulsion, generally seen in epileptic patients.

Spelt

A tough and resilient species of wheat growing mainly in Europe.

Steroids

Numerous naturally occurring or synthetic fat soluble organic compounds including sterols, bile acids and hormones.

Topical

Applied on the surface of the skin.

Wheat Germ

It is the embryo of the wheat kernel. It is a rich source of vitamins B and is used as a food supplement.

Whitehead

A non-inflamed open pore in the skin containing sebum.

Zit

A synonym for a pimple.

References

1. Adebamowo CA et al., *High School Dietary Intake and Teenage Acne*. Journal of the American Academy of Dermatology, Feb 2005; 52 : (2) 207-214
2. Fu,YJ; Chen, LY; Zu YG et al., *The Antibacterial Bacterial Activity of Clove Essential Oil Against Propionibacterium acnes and its Mechanism of Action*. Arch Dermatol 2009 Jan; 145(1) : 86-88
3. Smith RN, Mann NJ, Braue A, Makelainen H, Varigos GA. *A low-glycemic-load diet improves symptoms in acne vulgaris patients: a randomized controlled trial* Am J Clin Nutr July 2007; 86(1) : 107-15
4. Weber G, Adamczyk A, Freytag S. *Treatment of Acne with a Yeast Preparation*. Forts Chr Med Journal 1989
5. R Greenwood, P B Fenwick, and W J Cuncliffe. *Acne and anticonvulsants* Br Med J (Clin Res Ed) 1983 December 3; 287(6406) : 1669-1670
6. Chan HH, Wing Y, Su R. Van Krevel C, Lee S. *A control study of the cutaneous side effects of chronic lithium therapy* J Affect Disorder 2000 Jan-Mar; 57(1-3) : 107-13.

7. Bataille V, Sneider H, MacGregor AJ, SasieniP, Spector TD. *The influence of Genetics and Environmental Factors in the Pathogenesis of Acne: A Twin Study Of Acne in Women* Journal of Investigative Dermatology (2002)119 : 1317- 1322

8. Herane Maria, Ando Iwao *Acne in Infancy and Acne Genetics* Dermatology 2003;206 24-28

9. Ballanger F, Baudry P, N'Guyen JM Khammari A, Dreno B *Prevalence, Severity and Severity Risk Factors of Acne in High School Pupils: A Community –Based Study* Dermatology 2006; 212: 145-149

10. Tehrani R, Dharmalingam M. *Management of premenstrual acne with Cox-2 inhibitors; A placebo controlled study.* Indian J Dermatol Venereol Leprol 2004; 70 : 345-8

11. Schafer,T., Nienhaus, A., Vieluf, D., Berger, J. and Ring, J. (2001), *Epidemiology of acne in the general population: the risk of smoking.* British Journal of Dermatology, 145 : 100-104

12. Yosipovitch Gil, Tang Mark, Dawn Aerlyn G., Chen Mark, Goh Chee Leok, Chan Yiong Huak, Seng Lim Fong, *Study of Psychological Stress, Sebum Production and Acne Vulgaris in Adolescents* Acta Dermato-Venereologica March 2007 : 87(2) : 135-39

13. Hassanzadeh P, Bahmani M, Mehrabani D. *Bacterial resistance to antibiotics in acne vulgaris: An in vitro study.* Indian J Dermatol 2008; 53 : 122-4

14. Shalita, A. R., Smith, J. G., Parish, L.C., Sofman, M. S., and Chalker, D. K. (1995) Topical *Nicotinamide compared with Clyndamycin Gel in the treatment of inflammatory acne vulgaris.* International Journal of Dermatology, 34 : 434-37
15. Mills, O. H., Kligman, A. M., Pochi, P. and Comite, H. (1986), *Comparing 2.5%, %%, and 10% Benzoyl Peroxide on Inflammatory Acne Vulgaris.* International Journal of Dermatology, 25: 664-667
16. Lloyd J. R., *The use of microdermabrasion for acne: a pilot study* Dermatol Surg. 2001 April; 27(4) : 329-31
17. Harper Julie C., *Hormonal Therapy for Acne Using Oral Contraceptive Pills.* Seminars in Cutaneous Medicine and Surgery, June 2005 24 : (2) : 103-106
18. Verbov, J., (1976), *The place of intralesional steroid therapy in dermatology.* British Journal of Dermatology, 94: 1-57
19. Mahajan BB, Garg G. *Therapeutic efficacy of intralesional triamcinolone acetonide versus intralesional triamcinolone acetonide plus lincomycin in the treatment of nodulocystic acne.* Indian J Dermatol Venereol Leprol 2003; 69 : 217-9
20. Kawada A, Aragane Y, Kameyama H, Sangen Y, Tezuka T. *Acne Phototherapy with a high-intensity enhanced narrow-band blue light source: an open study and in vitro investigation.* J. Dermatol. Sc. 2002 Nov; 30(2) : 129-35

21. Papageorgiou P., Katsambas A., and Chu A., *Phototherapy with blue (415 nm) and red (660 nm) light in the treatment of acne vulgaris.* British Journal of Dermatology 2000; 142: 973-978
22. Leyden JJ, Shalita A, Thiboutot D, Washenik K, Webster G. *Topical retinoids in inflammatory acne: a retrospective, investigator-blinded, vehicle controlled, photographic assessment.* Clin Ther. 2005 Feb; 27(2) : 216-24
23. Shahidullah, M., Tham S. N. and Goh, C. –L. (1994) *Isotretinoin Therapy in Acne Vulgaris: A 10-Year Retrospective Study In Singapore.* International Journal of Dermatology, 33 : 60-63
24. Zander E, Weisman S. *Treatment of acne vulgaris with salicylic acid pads.* Clin. Ther. 1992 Mar-Apr; 14(2) : 247-53
25. Lee, H.-S, and Kim, I-H. (2003), *Salicylic Acid Peels for the Treatment of Acne Vulgaris in Asian Patients.* Dermatologic Surgery, 29 : 1196-1199
26. Wilkinson, R. D., Adam, J. E., Murray, J. J., Craig, Gibson E., *Benzoyl Peroxide and Sulfur: Foundation for Acne Management.* Canad. Med. Ass. J. July 1966 95 : 28-29
27. Harlen SL. *Steroid acne and rebound phenomenon* J Drugs Dermatol 2008 Jun; 7(6) : 547-50
28. Sule RR, Athavale NV, Gharpuray MB. *Lupus miliaris disseminatus faciei report of 4 cases.* Indian J Dermatol Venereol Leprol 1992; 58 : 102-4

29. Jacyk W. K. *Acne Vulgaris. Grades of Severity and Treatment Options.* SA Fam Pract 2003; 45(9) : 32-36

30. Jungfer, B., Janser, T., Przybilla, B., Plewig, G. *Solid Persistent Facial Edema of Acne: Successful Treatment with Isotretinoin and Ketotifen* Dermatology 1993; 187(1) : 34-37

31. Kilinc I, Gencoglan g, Inanir I, Dereli T. *Solid Facial Edema of Acne: failure of treatment with isotretinoin.* Eur J Dermatol. 2003 Sep-Oct; 13(5) : 503-4

32. Smith R, Mann N, Makelainen H, Roper J, Braue A, Varigos G. *A pilot study to determine the short term effects of a low glycemic load diet on hormonal markers of acne: a nonrandomized, parallel controlled feeding trial.* Mol Nutr Food Res 2008 Jun; 52(6) : 718-26

33. Slayden SM, Moran C, Sams WM Jr, Boots LR, Azziz R. *Hyperandrogenemia in patients presenting with acne.* Fertil. Steril 2001 May; 75(5) : 889-92.

34. Cordain L, Lindeberg S, Hurtado M, Hill K, Eaton SB, Brand-Miller J. *Acne Vulgaris: A Disease of Western Civilization* Arch Dermatol. 2002; 188(12) : 1584-1590.

35. Stamatiadis, D., Bulteau-Portois, M.-C. and Mowszowicz, I. (1988), *Inhibition of 5 ∞-reductase activity in human skin by zinc and azelaic acid.* British Journal of Dermatology, 119 : 627-632.

36. Meynadier J. *Efficacy and safety study of two zinc gluconate regimens in the treatment of inflammatory acne.* Eur. J Dermatol. 2000 Jun; 10(4) : 269-73

37. Costa Adilson, Lage Denise, Moises Thais Abdalla. *Acne and Diet: truth or myth?* An Bras Dermatol. 2010(8) : 346-353
38. Danby, F. William. *Acne and milk, the diet myth and beyond.* J Am Acad Dermatol 2005; 52 : 360-62

Books
1. James E. Fulton, *Acme RX*
2. *Occupational, Industrial and Environmental Toxicology* by Michael I. Greenberg 32; 339

Websites
www.hormonehelpny.com
www.umm.edu
www. nlm.nih.gov
http://blackhealthmatters.org
www.rosacea.org
www.bad.org.uk
www.dermnet.nz.org
www.skincarephysicians.com
www.wikipedia.org
www.wlnaturalhealth.com
www.thefreedictionary.com